M000287050

The

HCG DIET

Gourmet Cookbook

Volume 2

TAMMY SKYE

150 <u>MORE</u> Easy and Delicious Recipes
for the HCG Phase

© 2011 Tammy Skye/T Skye Enterprises Inc.

All Rights Reserved

ISBN - 978-0-9843999-2-5

Cover art Mitch Franklin
Cover and interior design Shadow Oak Studio

This book is copyrighted by the author and reproduction or distribution of this material is strictly prohibited in any form without written permission from the author except as permitted under Section 107 or 108 of the 1976 United States Copyright Act. The HCG Diet Gourmet Cookbook® is a registered trademark for the HCG Diet Gourmet Cookbook Series All Rights Reserved

If you have a clinic with an HCG program, an HCG blog, health website, or bookstore, become an affiliate or wholesale distributor of the HCG Diet Gourmet Cookbook series. To post a link on your website or inquire about wholesale opportunities, contact us at **affiliates@hcgrecipes.com**.

Disclaimer: This book is not intended to treat or diagnose any medical conditions. Anyone considering this diet should check with their doctor or healthcare provider before beginning this or any other weight loss program. The author assumes no responsibility for the use or misuse of the information in this book. Anyone following the HCG Diet or implementing the information provided in this book does so at their own risk. The author is not a medical doctor, is not qualified to treat any health conditions, and this book is not intended to provide individual medical advice in any form. It is recommended to seek care from a physician or healthcare provider before choosing to participate in the HCG Diet or any other medical weight loss protocol. Do not discontinue any medications without supervision from your physician. Individual HCG Diet weight loss results will vary.

FDA required statement: The FDA has not approved the use of HCG for weight loss and reports no evidence that HCG is effective for the treatment of obesity.

Scan the code below with your smartphone for further info, updates, discounts, and more or go to www.hcgrecipes.com.

Acknowledgments

This book is dedicated to all the HCG Dieters out there. I wish you amazing success and good health. I believe that with the HCG Diet, you have found the answer to your weight loss challenges and are well on your way to a slimmer body and healthier life. Much appreciation to Dr. A.T.W. Simeons, M.D., the founder of this program, and to Kevin Trudeau for his part in bringing this diet to the public.

There are far too many people to list here for their part in helping this book come to fruition, but I'd like to express my gratitude and thank a few special people and my team. Lori for her creative eye and tireless optimism in the design of this book. Cindy for her solid advice along the way and Wendy, Dave, Lisa, Nita, and Barbara for their honesty, feedback, time, and contribution. Special thanks to my father, Garry, and supportive family and friends.

I'd especially like to acknowledge the physicians and HCG Diet professionals who recommend this cookbook and who are dedicated to helping dieters achieve lasting success. And most of all I'd like to thank you... the reader of this book. Know that I am here, in spirit, supporting you and cheering you on as you embark on one of the most amazing weight loss journeys of your life.

Tammy Skye

Tammy Skye

To accomplish great things, we must not only act, but also dream: not only plan, but also believe.

— ANATOLE FRANCE

Table of Contents – Volume 2

Preface

Some of you may have read my personal story and experience with the HCG Diet in my first book, "The HCG Diet Gourmet Cookbook Volume 1," and how this diet has changed my life and my health. I really poured my heart out as I wrote "My Story." It was a somewhat painful and cathartic experience to share my very intimate and personal struggle to lose weight and the challenges I faced through my childhood, teen years, and adult life as an overweight woman. The death of my mother from complications of diabetes was a serious wake up call to examine my own health and lifestyle. It was when I reached the brink of weighing 200 pounds and felt the most helpless and hopeless in my struggle that I discovered the HCG Diet. Today, after several years, I'm maintaining my weight and enjoying life to the fullest.

I know the struggles many of you face trying to lose weight. The physical and emotional reasons behind why the weight gain occurred and has continued are extremely varied and personal to you. Some of the readers of this book may only need to lose 30 pounds while others may have 50, 100 pounds, or more to lose. Some may want to lose weight after having a baby or just want to feel comfortable in a bathing suit again. For some of you, losing weight has been a constant battle, for others, a sudden weight loss ultimatum that has very real consequences to your health and quality of life. Whatever your own personal reasons for losing weight and choosing this diet, I've done my very best with this book to offer you every tip, trick, tool, and bit of information I could think of to address your needs and questions, and help you be successful.

Many of you, like me, have tried just about every diet plan, pill, and promise over the years and rarely had lasting success. I tried the shakes, bars, supplements, and every fad and low calorie diet imaginable, without real or lasting results. The weight always came back — and more — and I was often drained of energy, hungry, and irritable the entire time. Then I discovered the HCG Diet and was absolutely amazed at the changes to my body, my metabolism, and my health. I won't say that this diet was easy and there were certainly challenges, fluctuations, and pitfalls along the way, but the lasting weight loss results made it all worth it in the end. I want to be there to encourage and support you through this process and share with you the life changing results that I know are possible for you with this diet.

This new *HCG Phase* (also known as Phase 2 or P2) Diet Gourmet Cookbook is far more than just recipes, and it offers the same solid foundation of information on the HCG Diet found in my first cookbook, as well as new and updated content and 150 more delicious recipes. It was my intention in writing this book that it stand on its own, be different from my first book, and still provide everything an HCG Dieter needs to be successful while observing the limited ingredients and restrictions of the original protocol of Dr. Simeons' HCG Diet. The 150 HCG Diet Gourmet Recipes in this book include the addition of some egg and cheese vegetarian dishes that will offer even more variety to the protocol as an occasional substitute for the more traditionally recommended proteins on the HCG Diet.

Some of the new information offered in this cookbook is based on my own personal experience, and much of it was gathered from conversations and questions from other HCG Dieters over the last few years. I felt a strong desire to share with you what I've learned about stabilizing and maintaining weight loss after the HCG Diet is over. In this new cookbook, I have a section on what foods to eat, how to stabilize your weight, sample menus, and guidance and advice on how to transition into the *Maintenance Phase*. Many dieters have shared with me how they fluctuate and have even gained weight after the diet is over and I've observed some common themes both with my own challenges over the years and their questions. During the last few years I've continued researching what works and what doesn't, and what factors and foods help people stabilize and maintain their weight loss.

This new cookbook also addresses the issue of mindset. As you face the future and the changes occurring in your body with the rapid weight loss you are experiencing, it is important to allow yourself to change mentally as well. As I went through this process myself, I learned a lot about what my emotional triggers are in my relationship to food and my weight. This book offers some sound advice on how to make this shift in mindset and lifestyle to help you adjust to the new you and how to make these changes at a rate that is comfortable for you.

Overall, the best advice I can offer as you lose weight following the HCG Diet program is to become more aware and take daily steps toward good health. When you move into the *Maintenance Phase*, consider switching to a whole food-based diet and eating more fruits and vegetables. Cut down on sugar or start gradually replacing it with Stevia or natural sugars like raw honey. Over time you will find that your tastes change and you start to crave nutritious, healthy foods over cookies and sodas. You will find yourself with increased energy and easily able to maintain your weight loss. The HCG Diet is not so much a "diet" as a corrective procedure that helps you STOP "dieting" for good.

Please don't feel like you have to change your lifestyle overnight. I make many recommendations for health and lifestyle changes within this book, and much of my focus is getting back to "real food," a true "whole food" diet. I have to admit that the process of change was a gradual one in my own life. I didn't just give up diet soda and sugar and start drinking green drinks and eating organic overnight. It was a gradual shift toward health and it took a while to get there.

I know that the HCG Diet can create an incredible transformation in your body and your life as you now have the tools and the means to finally lose the weight and keep it off for good. I strongly urge you to make a commitment to yourself right now to stick with the diet, stay positive and on track, and look toward the future: your future as the slim, healthy, vibrant, energetic person that you know you can be. I wish you all the best as you go on this amazing weight loss journey with the HCG Diet.

To help you be successful with your weight loss, I'd like to share some special free gifts with you. You can access these Free HCG Diet tools at http://pages.hcgrecipes. com/Secret-stash-5. I wish you all the best as you go on this amazing weight loss journey with the HCG Diet.

Enjoy the recipes!

Tammy Skye

Our bodies are our gardens
- our wills are our gardeners.
— WILLIAM SHAKESPEARE

Special Offer to Readers...

IF YOU ENJOY THE RECIPES IN THIS BOOK, YOU'RE GONNA LOVE THIS FREE GIFT!
CLAIM $147 OF MORE HCG DIET RECIPES AND EXTRA DIET SUPPORT

❑ Yes, I enjoyed my HCG Diet Gourmet Cookbook and would like to receive my
   HCG Diet Support Package, Including:
- The Phase 3 Quick Start Guide — A $37.00 value
- A digital copy of Pounds and Inches Recipes (The original plan by Dr. A.T.W. Simeons with
  recipes from the HCG Diet Gourmet Cookbook Series) — A $9.97 value
- A Full Round (43 Days) of daily email support messages to help you be successful. — A $75.00 value
- Audio Q & A with Tammy Skye answering your most pressing and important HCG Diet
  Questions — A $25.00 Value

GET THE SUPPORT YOU NEED — just cover S&H of $14.95.

There is a one time charge of $14.95 for your HCG Diet Support Package materials. We wish
you all the best on every phase of the diet and want to be here to help you to achieve your best
results and weight loss success. Please email us at support@hcgrecipes.com if you have any
questions about our products or services.

I know you're going to enjoy your HCG Diet Gourmet Cookbook and the Delicious recipes. In
Good Health!

Name_____

Address_____

City_____ State _____ Country _____

Email address _____

Credit Card ❑ Visa ❑ Mastercard ❑ AMEX ❑ Discover

Credit Card Number _____ Exp. Date _____ 3 digit code _____

Signature _____ Date _____

Fax 1-855-HCG-COOK or Sign up at www.hcgrecipes.com/FreeGift2

Disclaimer: The information in HCG Diet Gourmet Cookbook and HCGRecipes.com is not intended to treat or diagnose any medical conditions
and we encourage you to seek support and and health care from your physician. Anyone considering this diet should check with their doctor or
healthcare provider before beginning this or any other weight loss program. HCGRecipes and its affiliates assume no responsibility for the use
or misuse of information provided and while we offer general information and emotional support, we are not qualified to offer medical advice
and defer to the client's healthcare provider. Anyone following the HCG Diet protocol or implementing our services does so at their own risk.
It is recommended to seek care from a physician or healthcare provider before and while choosing to participate in the HCG Diet or any other
medical weight loss protocol. Do not discontinue any medications without supervision from your physician. Individual HCG Diet weight loss
results will vary.

FDA required statement: The FDA has not approved the use of HCG for weight loss and reports no evidence that HCG is effective for the
treatment of obesity.

HCG Diet Terms and Abbreviations

HCG — Human Chorionic Gonadotropin. A natural medication often used as a fertility treatment; researched and developed for the HCG Diet Protocol for weight loss by Dr. A.T.W. Simeons.

HHCG — Homeopathic HCG.

LIW — Last Injection Weight. The weight recorded on the last day of HCG injection. Used to monitor weight during Phase 3 (*Stabilization Phase*).

LSDW — Last Sublingual Dose Weight. The weight recorded on the last day of HCG sublingual dosage.

VLCD — Very Low Calorie Diet. The term used to describe the 500 calorie *HCG Phase* of the diet.

IU — International Unit. A term that identifies the dosage of a medication (for example, the amount of HCG taken daily during the *HCG Phase* of the diet is 125-200 IU).

SL — Sublingual. Placing a medication under the tongue where it is absorbed by the capillaries and into the bloodstream. HCG can be taken this way as an alternative to injections.

SC/SQ — Subcutaneous. Injecting a medication just under the skin rather than into the muscle.

IM — Intramuscular. Injecting a medication into the muscle.

R1 — **(Round 1), R2 (Round 2),** etc. An abbreviation to identify a specific round of HCG. Helpful when there is a lot of weight to lose and multiple rounds are undertaken.

Loading — The term to describe the first two days on the HCG when it is required to eat large amounts of high fat foods in preparation for the Very Low Calorie Diet.

Nutritional Loading — Eating very healthy foods and supplements before and after the *HCG Phase* (Phase 2 or P2) to promote optimal health.

Prep and Load — (Phase 1 or P1) Preparing for the HCG Diet and loading properly before beginning the *HCG Phase* of the diet.

(continued)

The HCG Phase — (Phase 2 or P2) The use of HCG in combination with a Very Low Calorie Diet (500 calories per day).

The Stabilization Phase — (Phase 3 or P3) The 3 week period of a varied, normal calorie diet with the exception of starch and sugar.

The Maintenance Phase — (Phase 4 or P4) The last phase of the diet where carbohydrates are gradually incorporated back into the diet and weight loss is maintained for life.

Immunity —When the HCG is no longer effective and a break from the diet is needed. Symptoms are severe hunger, weakness, fatigue, and mental fogginess.

Apple Day — A technique recommended by Dr. Simeons to break up a plateau in the *HCG Phase* of the diet. After a plateau of 4 or more days, eat 6 apples during that day while drinking minimal water. Weight loss should resume the following day.

Steak Day — A technique used if a weight gain of 2 pounds over LIW/LSDW occurs during the *Stabilization Phase* (Phase 3 or P3). The dieter must perform a Steak Day on the same day as the gain and eat nothing until the evening and then eat a large steak with either a large apple or raw tomato. The weight gain should be corrected by the following day.

About the HCG Diet

What is the HCG Diet?

The HCG Diet is a revolutionary diet using HCG or Human Chorionic Gonadotropin combined with a low calorie diet of 500 calories a day. Taking HCG for a period of 23 to 43 days while observing a strict, food specific, low calorie diet allows the body to burn fat at a rapid rate. While the dieter is on the HCG, the body utilizes the abnormal fat stores of the body for fuel. It is also theorized by the doctor who developed the diet that the hypothalamus gland is reset at the end of the protocol, improving metabolism and regulating the endocrine system more efficiently. After the *HCG Phase* (also known as Phase 2 or P2), you can eat a normal calorie diet with a large variety of foods, with the exception of starches and sugars, for a period of 3 weeks that I call the *Stabilization Phase* (also known as Phase 3 or P3). Finally, in the *Maintenance Phase* (also known as Phase 4 or P4), you can begin to slowly incorporate carbohydrates back into your diet and enjoy your new, faster metabolism.

History of the HCG Diet

The HCG Diet protocol was developed by Dr. A.T.W. Simeons, M.D. in the 1950s when he discovered the connection between obesity and a treatment using HCG for boys who had hormonal imbalances and were significantly overweight. He theorized and studied the use of HCG as a treatment for weight loss and found it extremely effective when used properly, by correcting a metabolic disorder of the hypothalamus gland. His patients lost incredible amounts of weight and had an improved metabolism as a result of the treatment. I highly recommend reading the original book by Dr. A.T.W. Simeons, *"Pounds and Inches"* for a detailed analysis of the process and how it affects the body. A copy can be found on my website at www.hcgrecipes.com.

The HCG Diet experienced a resurgence since the 2007 release of Kevin Trudeau's book, "The Weight Loss Cure They Don't Want You to Know About," which discusses in detail Dr. Simeons' original protocol with a few minor variations and other health recommendations and suggestions. The differences between Kevin Trudeau's version of the HCG Diet program and Dr. Simeons' are that Mr. Trudeau omits the use of shellfish in the diet, breadsticks, and also the orange as a fruit choice. Otherwise, the diet is virtually the same. The recipes in this book follow the original HCG Diet developed by Dr. Simeons and do contain oranges and shellfish but can be easily modified to substitute white fish, beef or chicken, if desired.

Expected Weight Loss

Weight loss of up to one pound a day can be expected. Women tend to lose a half pound per day on average, and the average daily weight loss for men is slightly higher. The amount you can lose also depends on how much you have to lose and how strictly you follow the diet. If you want to lose 100 pounds or more, you will lose more and faster than if you only have 20 pounds to lose. It is advisable to stop the diet if more than 34 pounds have been lost in one round or if 43 injections have been completed. People who have a lot of weight to lose can safely lose a little more, if desired, but it is advisable to transition to the *Stabilization Phase* (Phase 3 or P3) when 34 pounds is reached.

Choosing a Clinic

The dosages for injections should be 125-200 IU of HCG taken once per day (a higher dosage of 125-166 IU twice a day is recommended for sublingual formulations) 7 days a week for a period of 23 days, or 6 days a week for a 43 day round. Note: Many dieters report that taking the maximum dosage of 200 IU's or higher may actually stall weight loss and even increase hunger. The food choices and other restrictions should be compliant with the original protocol. You should not be required to purchase any additional supplements or shakes, or be advised to use oils on your body while on the *HCG Phase* of the program. This can slow or stall your weight loss and can often be a costly and unnecessary expense. In cases of severe dryness or cracking, mineral oil can be used topically and won't stall weight loss as other oils ingested or applied to the skin will.

It is very important to choose a reputable clinic and physician to monitor you while on the program and make sure that your HCG is fresh and potent at the time you begin. When evaluating a clinic for their HCG program, consider the cost, support, and benefits they offer you. Although not officially endorsed by the FDA for weight loss, HCG is an all natural prescription medication that an open-minded doctor can prescribe for you, and HCG is available at most pharmacies.

Multiple Rounds of HCG

If you require more than one round to reach your goal weight, you can begin another round after a period of about 6 weeks, including 3 weeks on the *Stabilization Phase* (Phase 3 or P3) and 3 weeks (or more) of *Maintenance Phase* eating. You should increase the time between rounds after 2 or more rounds in order to prevent immunity. By following this plan and taking breaks between rounds, it's quite possible to lose 100 pounds or more in a year.

Immunity

Immunity to HCG can sometimes occur and is characterized by extreme hunger and feelings of weakness and lightheadedness. This is an indication that you should consider transitioning to the *Stabilization Phase* (Phase 3 or P3) and to take a break. Another time you might experience immunity is when you get close to your goal weight or the ideal weight for you. To prevent immunity, it is helpful and recommended by Dr. Simeons to take one day off per week when doing a full 43 day course. If you feel you are having the symptoms of immunity, you should increase your food intake from 500 to 800 calories per day, and continue to eat *HCG Phase* allowed foods. You must complete a minimum of 23 days of injections before transitioning to the *Stabilization Phase* (Phase 3 or P3). The HCG will not allow you to reduce your weight below a natural, healthy level without showing you signs of immunity so it is wise to take a break if you begin experiencing the symptoms. If you want that starved, gaunt, skinny look, this is not the diet for you. The HCG Diet will, however, help you achieve a normal, healthy weight for your age, height, and frame.

Exercise

It isn't recommended to exercise heavily while on the *HCG Phase* of the diet. Heavy exercise seems to cause stalls in weight loss, possibly due to the water retention required by muscles during exercise. Light exercise like walking, yoga, stretching, and rebounding are good exercises to do. Once you transition to Phase 3, you can start your cardiovascular, weight lifting, and regular exercise routine if you wish.

The Abnormal Fat Loss Phenomenon

One phenomenon experienced by most HCG Dieters following Dr. Simeons' protocol is the way the HCG tends to redistribute fat away from your "problem areas" or abnormal fat deposits. In my personal experience, I noticed that my hips and thighs lost the highest percentage

of inches, as well as significant inches lost from my stomach and waist. This phenomenon is fairly unique to the HCG Diet when compared with other weight loss programs.

Ways to Take HCG

INJECTIONS

HCG is most commonly injected intramuscularly (IM), but some people inject subcutaneously (SC/SQ). The recommended dosage is 125 IU up to 200 IU injected daily, 6 days per week for a period of 43 days or daily for a period of 23 days. It is not advisable to go higher than 200 IU daily or weight gain may occur. The HCG must be kept cold, dark, and fresh. It can last in the refrigerator and remain effective for 2-3 weeks.

SUBLINGUAL HCG

The sublingual form (SL) of the HCG Diet has become popular among dieters who are enjoying the same weight loss success as those who are injecting the HCG. Most clinics have their own proprietary formula with the saline base. When taking sublingual HCG, it is necessary to take a stronger dosage (150-166 IU) under the tongue twice a day (morning and evening) in order to ensure receiving an adequate dosage. Some clinics report that it is not necessary to take the breaks between rounds when using sublingual HCG, but I strongly recommend taking them anyway. The *HCG Phase* (Phase 2 or P2) is so restrictive that even if you don't experience immunity, you still need the varied nutrition and breaks to give your body a rest and ensure good health.

HOMEOPATHIC HCG

Homeopathic HCG (HHCG) products were available at one time. I have not personally tried these products and there are no studies at this time showing whether they are as effective as using the natural HCG. Many dieters have reported good success and lasting results using the HHCG products. Homeopathic HCG products are taken sublingually under the tongue and dieters must avoid all use of mint when using HHCG because it is believed to interfere with its effectiveness. Finding reliable HHCG products has been a challenge for dieters and there have been issues with HHCG manufacture, labeling, ingredients, and current FDA regulations. Many HHCG products have been discontinued and removed from circulation.

The Four Phases of the HCG Diet

There are four steps or Phases of the HCG Diet. The first is "**Prep and Load**" (also known as Phase 1 or P1). The second is the *HCG Phase* (also known as Phase 2 or P2). The third is the *Stabilization Phase* (also known as Phase 3 or P3), and the fourth is the *Maintenance Phase* (also known as Phase 4 or P4).

Prep and Load
CLEANSING

Consider a period of detoxification and cleansing prior to beginning the HCG Diet. Performing colon cleanses, candida cleansing, and taking additional vitamin and mineral supplements to prepare the body for the diet can maximize weight loss and improve overall health. It is important to give your body high quality, nutritious foods and supplements before and after the strict *HCG Phase* of the diet. Consider daily or occasional vegetable juicing during this time to provide extra healthy nutrients and energy. Many people have found that cleansing and detoxing prior to beginning the diet can substantially help maximize the benefit of the HCG Diet and assist with successful maintenance.

NUTRITIONAL LOADING

I highly recommend what I call "Nutritional Loading" before and after the *HCG Phase* of the diet, which essentially means taking quality supplements, a green drink, trace minerals, and eating high quality, healthy food including lots of fruits and vegetables. Taking supplements during the *HCG Phase* is not recommended by Dr. Simeons as it may slow or stall weight loss, so it is important to build up the body's systems before and after for optimal health.

MENTAL PREPARATION

Prepare yourself mentally by committing to stick to the program. Clean out your cupboards and throw out or donate any food that could tempt you while on the diet. Take some before, during, and after pictures to help you stay motivated while on the diet, as well as accurate body measurements, so you can track your progress along the way. Buy yourself an accurate digital food scale for preparing your meals and consider a new digital bathroom scale if you need one. A scale that measures your weight in .2 pound increments is best. During times of slower weight loss, that .2 pound loss can help you stay motivated.

As you prepare for this diet, focus on your goals and list in your journal all the reasons you want to lose weight. Think about your health, your family, and all the ways losing the weight will change your life. Visualize yourself at your goal weight, buying new clothes, and feeling slim and healthy. Remember that you do not have to do this diet alone. Consider joining an HCG support group, and prepare your family and friends to support you in your weight loss journey.

2 DAYS OF FAT LOADING

For the first two days of the program, while taking the HCG, it is important to "load" by eating high fat foods. This is an absolutely essential phase where you must eat a high calorie, high fat diet. Oils, cheeses, avocados, nuts, pastries, cream, fatty meats, and other rich foods are recommended for these two loading days.

It is very important not to skip this phase. It is an absolutely necessary part of the diet. People who have skipped this step have reported being excessively hungry for the first week or two of the low calorie *HCG Phase* of the diet. It is not a particularly pleasant experience to eat the sheer volume of high fat food, especially when you aren't used to it. Just do the best you can and don't hold back. Consider eating smaller amounts of high fat food every hour rather than large amounts of food at one sitting. Focusing on concentrated high fat food over carbohydrates will give you the best results. As a result of loading properly, you should experience little to no hunger when you transition to the 500 calorie limit of the *HCG Phase* of the diet.

The HCG Phase

During the *HCG Phase* (Phase 2 or P2) of the diet, the dieter takes injections (once a day) of 125-200 IU doses of HCG daily or 150 IU SL HCG (twice a day) for a period of 23-43 days while observing a very specific, low-fat, 500 calorie diet. The food choices are very limited and specific and must be adhered to strictly in order for the diet to be successful. A list of allowable foods is provided for you in a later section of the book, along with some per serving calorie counts to help keep your total calories for the day below 500.

During the *HCG Phase* it is important to avoid contact with all external fats such as creams and lotions. Dr. Simeons found that even trace amounts of externally applied oils could stall the weight loss process. Only powdered makeup, lipstick, and eye pencil may be used. In cases of severe dryness or cracking, a small amount of mineral oil or aloe vera juice can be used on problem areas.

PLATEAUS

Plateaus are normal with this diet. Weight loss usually occurs in a stair step fashion with a consistent large drop in weight followed by a slight plateau or slower losses for a few days. At least one significant plateau occurs in the second half of the protocol that often lasts 4-6 days. This is normal and will resolve itself in time so don't be alarmed when this happens. If a plateau continues longer than 4 days, an "Apple Day" can be considered.

THE APPLE DAY

Although most plateaus will resolve naturally on their own, it can be very discouraging to experience several days without weight loss. An "Apple Day" can be used when a dieter reaches a plateau (no loss for a period of 4-5 days). The way to do an Apple Day is to eat 6 apples over a 24 hour period and drink **minimal water** — just enough to quench your thirst. This usually resolves the plateau, and regular weight loss normally resumes the next morning.

The Stabilization Phase

The *Stabilization Phase* (Phase 3 or P3) is a three week period following the *HCG Phase* where you are allowed and encouraged to eat normal amounts of food and calories with the exception of starches and sugars. It is an important part of this diet protocol as it is the period where the weight and metabolism stabilize at a new, higher metabolic set point.

For the first week or two on the *Stabilization Phase* you can expect wild fluctuations in your weight. This is normal and your weight will stabilize at some point during the three weeks. A glass of wine, beer, or other alcohol can be enjoyed on P3 without issue, as well as a more varied and exciting diet. It is important for HCG Dieters to weigh themselves daily on P3 and immediately do a "Steak Day" if a gain of over 2 pounds of your LIW (last injection weight) occurs.

THE STEAK DAY

A "Steak Day" is done if a gain of over two pounds occurs after the morning weighing. To do a Steak Day, all food must be avoided throughout the day (water is fine) and then a large steak and either a raw apple or raw tomato must be consumed. The steak can be prepared with a variety of spices, but no salt. Doing a Steak Day will usually correct the weight gain by the following morning and you can resume your regular Phase 3 stabilizing diet. The Steak Day must be done the same day you notice the 2 pound gain. It is an important part of this phase of the diet and is critical to stabilizing the weight and resetting the metabolism.

When you reach the end of the *HCG Phase* (Phase 2 or P2), it is time to transition into the *Stabilization Phase* of the HCG Diet. This is a critical aspect of the diet and is the time when your body and weight stabilize and your new and faster metabolism kicks in. After your last dose of HCG, continue to observe the low calorie diet for 72 hours as the HCG leaves your system. You will now increase your calories to a normal amount and enjoy a wider variety of foods as long as they are free of starch and sugar. The calories will vary per individual depending on height, weight, and activity level.

For women, it is usually approximately 1700-2500 calories per day and for men, 2200-2700 calories per day. It is important to start immediately eating normal calorie amounts and foods rather than continuing to diet and just doubling your portions. Many dieters feel apprehensive about eating more fat and calories and yet this is very important to stabilizing properly.

Again, during the first few days and weeks on the *Stabilization Phase*, you can expect some wild swings as your weight fluctuates and then begins to stabilize. Do a Steak Day if you go two pounds over your LIW, as needed, and continue to eat normal calories and foods thereafter.

The Maintenance Phase

The *Maintenance Phase* (Phase 4 or P4) involves gradually introducing starches and carbohydrates back into your diet. This is the transition back to "real life" and normal eating patterns. Even though you have likely met your weight loss goal, you should continue to monitor your weight daily. As you transition from the *Stabilization Phase* to the *Maintenance Phase* and begin to introduce more carbohydrates back into your diet, you can be assured that your metabolism is significantly improved and your weight is stabilized. This is the healthy eating plan that you will enjoy for the rest of your life.

When choosing foods for a long term maintenance diet, I highly recommend that all foods eaten during Maintenance be as organic and unprocessed as possible.

When shopping for yourself and your family, choose wild caught fish and seafood, free-range and organic poultry and eggs, grass fed organic meats and dairy products, healthy fats, plenty of fruits and vegetables, and limit grains and starches to 2-3 servings per day. I also recommend "Nutritional Loading" by taking healthy supplements and a daily green drink, especially if you have multiple rounds to do and plan to go back on the *HCG Phase* to lose additional weight.

There really are very few restrictions on the *Maintenance Phase* as far as foods you can eat and you can have nearly any food in moderation.

Consistently choosing healthy, unprocessed foods and minimizing sugar and starch in your diet will help you achieve lasting success. It is very important to consider the kinds and quality of the foods you eat rather than focusing on the number of fat grams and calories. On the *Maintenance Phase*, drop the diet mentality and choose highly nutritious foods that will energize you and keep you healthy.

HCG DIET Tip

During the Maintenance Phase, add kefir to fresh fruit smoothies. Kefir adds both a wonderful flavor and extra probiotics and protein.

HCG Phase Foods

Proteins

Proteins should be precisely 100 grams, weighed raw using an accurate food scale. You should have two servings per day at different meals and all visible fat must be removed prior to cooking.

Chicken breast (skinless)

Beef (lean beef, 7% fat or less)

Fresh white fish

Lobster

Crab

Shrimp

Nonfat cottage cheese (100 grams)

1 whole egg plus 3 egg whites

SPECIAL INSTRUCTIONS – PROTEINS

Chicken

Weighed raw to precisely 100 grams

Breast meat only

Skin and all fat removed

Ideally organic

Cooked without fat (may use chicken broth or water)

Beef

Weighed raw to precisely 100 grams

Very lean (7% fat or less) with all fat removed

Avoid marbling when choosing cuts of meat

Cooked without fat (may use beef broth or water)

Fish

Weighed raw to precisely 100 grams

Lean variety (avoid fatty fish such as tuna and salmon while on the *HCG Phase*)

Ideally wild caught

Skin removed

Shellfish

Weighed raw to precisely 100 grams (subtract 15-20 grams if using pre-cooked meat such as canned crab)

Cooked without fat (may use water or allowed vegetable broth)

Ideally wild caught

Avoid processed, cooked seafood items such as imitation crab due to additives and sugar

Cottage Cheese

Precisely 100 grams nonfat cottage cheese

Limit cottage cheese HCG Diet meals to 2-3 times per week due to the milk sugars which may stall weight loss if cottage cheese is eaten too frequently

Enjoy cottage cheese as an occasional vegetarian option

Eggs

1 whole egg, plus 3 egg whites

Enjoy eggs as an occasional vegetarian option

If a recipe calls for a partial egg serving (i.e. 1 egg white), make sure to eat the rest of the eggs to complete a full protein serving

Vegetables

Asparagus

Beet greens

Cabbage

Celery

Chard

Chicory

Cucumber

Fennel

Green salad

Onions

Radishes

Spinach

Tomatoes

H C G
D I E T
Tip *Carry baggies of chopped veggies or apple slices for an on-the-go snack or to enjoy if you get hungry.*

SPECIAL INSTRUCTIONS – VEGETABLES

Two vegetable servings per day at separate meals

Do not mix vegetables at the same meal

Enjoy vegetables in reasonable amounts; there is no restriction on the amount of vegetables you can eat per meal as long as you stay below the 500 calorie limit for the day

Prepare vegetables without fat or oils

Vary the vegetables you eat to maximize nutritional value

Fruits

1 apple

1 orange

1/2 grapefruit

Handful of strawberries

SPECIAL INSTRUCTIONS – FRUITS

Two servings of allowed fruits per day

Eat fruit servings at separate meals in recommended amounts

If a recipe calls for a partial fruit serving (i.e. 2 orange segments), make sure to eat the rest of the fruit for that meal to complete a full fruit serving

If you are prone to hunger, you may have a fruit serving for breakfast and save your second fruit serving for an evening snack

Miscellaneous Foods and Specialty Ingredients

Juice of 1 lemon daily

Spices (fresh or dried)

Two Melba toasts, breadsticks, or grissini (one per meal)

1 tablespoon of milk daily

Tea

Coffee

Mineral water

Bragg's liquid aminos

Apple cider vinegar (other sugar free vinegars)

Stevia (flavored, powdered, or liquid) or other natural calorie-free sweetener

Flavor drops

Chicken and Beef broth (using HCG Diet Broth is ideal but commercial broths are fine)

SPECIAL INSTRUCTIONS – MISCELLANEOUS FOODS AND SPECIALTY INGREDIENTS

Enjoy reasonable amounts of many of the foods on the list unless otherwise indicated

Watch for hidden sugars and starchy binders in ingredients like spices

Melba toast servings are not to be combined but eaten at separate meals

Eliminate Melba toast if you find your weight loss stalls

Reduce amount of Bragg's liquid aminos to control sodium content, if desired

Reduce sodium content of recipes when using commercial broth by substituting half water

Foods to Avoid

All foods other than those specifically recommended for the *HCG Phase*

Sugar

Artificial sweeteners

Artificial and chemical ingredients

Starchy additives

Fats and oils

Calorie Counts for the Foods on the HCG Diet

Values may vary slightly depending on cut or variety

PROTEINS

Chicken Breast: 100 grams = 25 grams of protein, 2 grams of fat, and 135 calories

White Fish: 100 grams = 25 grams of protein, 4 grams of fat, and 120 calories

Lean Beef: 100 grams = 25 grams of protein, 5-10 grams fat (depending on the cut), and 140 calories

Shrimp/Lobster/Crab: 100 grams = 25 grams of protein, 1.5 grams fat, and 100 calories

Eggs: 1 Whole Egg, plus 3 egg whites = 17 grams protein, 4 grams fat, 127 calories

Nonfat Cottage Cheese: 100 grams contains 17.5 grams protein, .5 grams fat, 85 calories

VEGETABLES

(These are approximate serving sizes. You may have more or less if you wish as long as you stay below 500 total calories for the day.)

Cabbage: 2 cups chopped = 1.5 grams protein, 0 grams fat, and 50 calories

Spinach: 2 cups chopped = 2 grams protein, 0 grams fat, and 25 calories

Tomatoes: 1 ½ cups chopped = 3 grams protein, 0 grams fat, 50 calories

Celery: 1 ½ cups chopped = 1 gram protein, 0 grams fat, 25 calories

Radishes: 8 medium radishes = 1 gram protein, 0 grams fat, 18 calories

Cucumber: 1 medium cucumber = 2 grams protein, 0 grams fat, 45 calories

Lettuce/Mixed Greens: 2 cups shredded = 0 protein, 0 fat, 10 calories

Asparagus: 1 ½ cups cooked = 5 grams protein, 0 fat, 60 calories

Fennel: 1 ½ cups cooked = 1 gram protein, 0 grams fat, 40 calories

Chicory: 1 cup raw = 1 gram protein, 0 grams fat, 15 calories

Calorie Counts for the Foods on the HCG Diet

Values may vary slightly depending on cut or variety

Beet Greens: 1 1/2 cups cook = 1 gram protein, 0 grams fat, 15 calories

Chard: 1 ½ cups cooked = 1 gram protein, 0 grams fat, 55 calories

Onions: full serving is 1/2 medium onion = .5 grams protein, 0 grams fat, 24 calories

FRUITS

Apples: 1 medium apple = .5 grams protein, 0 fat, 90 calories

Grapefruit: ½ grapefruit = 1 gram protein, 0 fat, 50 calories

Strawberries: 5 large strawberries = .5 grams protein, 0 fat, 30 calories

Oranges: 1 medium orange = 1 gram protein, 0 fat, 65 calories

MISCELLANEOUS AND SPECIALTY INGREDIENTS

Dried Spices: 1 pinch = 0 protein, 0 fat, less than 10 calories

Fresh Ginger: 1 tablespoon = 0 protein, 0 fat, less than 5 calories

Garlic: 1 clove garlic = 0 protein, 0 fat, less than 5 calories

Minced Onion: 1 tablespoon = 0 protein, 0 fat, less than 5 calories

Melba Toast: 1 Melba Toast = .5 grams protein, 0 fat, 18 calories

Bragg's Liquid Aminos: 1 dash = .5 grams protein, 0 fat, 0 calories

Apple Cider Vinegar: 1 tablespoon = 0 protein, 0 fat, 0 calories

Cayenne Pepper Sauce: 1 teaspoon = 0 protein, 0 fat, 0 calories

Fat-free Milk: 1 tablespoon = .2 grams protein, 0 fat, less than 5 calories

Lemon Juice: 1 ounce = 0 protein, 0 fat, 8 calories

Chicken Broth: 1 cup = 1.5 grams protein, 0-1 grams fat, 15 calories

Beef Broth: 1 cup = 1 gram protein, 0-1 grams fat, 10 calories

Stevia: 1 serving = 0 protein, 0 fat, 0 calories

Flavor Drops: 0 protein, 0 fat, 0 calories

Spices, Teas, and Specialty Ingredients

Spices

Spices are not only delicious but have many health benefits as well. I recommend organic spices and spice mixes as they are better for you and are less likely to have MSG added. Spices can be enjoyed fresh (the best option for many of the recipes) or dried.

Fresh onions and garlic (used in small amounts in many of the recipes in this cookbook)

Basil (fresh or dried)

Bay leaf

Black pepper

Cardamom

Cayenne pepper

Chili powder (traditional and varieties like Chipotle are used in the recipes)

Chives

Cilantro (fresh)

Cinnamon

Cloves

Cumin

Dill

Garlic

Ginger

Marjoram

Mint

Mustard powder

Nutmeg

Onion powder

Oregano

Parsley

Rosemary

Saffron

Sage

Tarragon

Thyme

Turmeric (primary ingredient in Curry)

Spice Mixes

Using various spice mixes is another way to simplify your HCG Diet cooking without having to purchase many of the spices individually. Just make certain to check for harmful or weight stalling ingredients like MSG and starchy additives, such as corn or food starch and sugar.

Italian herb mix

Cajun seasoning

Allspice

Chili powder spice mix

Curry spice mix

Garam masala (an Indian spice mix)

Poultry seasoning

Steak and seafood rubs

Health Benefits of Spices

- Anti-bacterial/anti-viral

- Anti-fungal

- Stimulate blood flow and circulation

- Anti-carcinogenic properties

- Detoxification (liver, heavy metals, candida, colon, and other cleansing properties)

- Clear the lungs and promote respiratory health

- Increase brain function

- Blood sugar control

- Aid in digestion

- Rich in antioxidants, phyto-nutrients, and trace minerals

- Anti-inflammatory properties

- Helpful for weight loss

- Strengthen the immune system

Teas and Coffee

OOLONG TEA

Also known as Wulong, oolong tea is a wonderful addition to any HCG Diet program. Not only is it believed to stimulate metabolism and weight loss, but it is also a soothing and mellow flavored beverage with antioxidants and other health benefits. It comes in caffeinated and decaffeinated forms and is a lovely alternative to a morning cup of coffee.

YERBA MATE

Yerba Mate is a tea grown and popularized originally in Argentina that has a strong, powerful flavor. It has been shown to promote weight loss and stimulate the metabolism as well as provide the body with antioxidants and other health benefits. It can be enjoyed hot or iced and is available in caffeinated and decaffeinated varieties. Traditionally, Yerba Mate is served steeped in hot water and slowly sipped through a special metal straw and seasoned Mate cup in Argentina. In the rest of the world it is conveniently available as a loose leaf or bagged tea.

GREEN TEA

Green tea has many health benefits and is believed to stimulate metabolism and promote weight loss. Full of antioxidants, drinking 1-3 cups a day is a wonderful addition to your HCG Diet program and a healthful habit for life. Green tea can be enjoyed caffeinated, decaffeinated, bagged, loose leafed, and in many flavored varieties. Enjoy Green tea hot or iced for a delicious and healthy treat throughout the day.

WHITE AND BLACK TEA

White and Black tea are essentially the same variety of leaves and it is the level of the oxidation and stronger flavor that is the primary distinction between the two. Teas can offer different flavors and properties depending on where they are grown. They contain antioxidants and health benefits and are available in caffeinated, decaffeinated, bagged, loose leaf, and flavored varieties.

HERBAL TEAS

Teas such as chamomile, rose hip, ginger, mint, and other herbal teas contain antioxidants and often have other health benefits such as aiding in digestion (ginger and peppermint), promoting relaxation, and stress relief.

COFFEE

Coffee is a permitted beverage while on the HCG Diet. It comes in many different varieties and roasts and often takes on different flavors and properties depending on where it is grown. Coffee can be enjoyed in a variety of ways while on the HCG Diet, from a strong espresso beverage to a traditional cup of coffee sweetened with Stevia or another calorie free natural sweetener. Enjoy your coffee while on the HCG Diet with Flavor drops or with the flavored liquid varieties of Stevia available.

Flavorings and Specialty Ingredients

STEVIA

Stevia is an all natural herb that has been used for centuries as a calorie free sweetener. It is grown primarily in South American countries and has been utilized in many beverages and food products in countries like Japan for many years. Stevia is now widely available as a calorie free sweetener/food supplement in many health stores and grocery stores across the country and is becoming more widely known as the natural sweetener of choice in the United States and Europe.

Stevia is many times sweeter than sugar in the powdered and liquid forms, so feel free to adjust your use of Stevia to taste in the recipes in this cookbook. I recommend choosing naturally processed, high quality brands for the best taste and sweetness. Stevia cooks well and is available as a liquid or a powder and is offered in many flavored varieties. You can even grow your own Stevia herbs in your garden and enjoy their natural sweetness when crushed and added to tea and other beverages. Try Stevia drizzled over fruit, added to entrees, salads, desserts, beverages, and baked dishes.

Note: While Stevia is preferred, Erythritol, Xylitol, and Vegetable glycerin (food grade) are other natural sweeteners allowed in moderation during the _HCG Phase_.

FLAVOR DROPS

Flavor drops are calorie free, oil free, sugar free, pure flavor essences made with mostly natural ingredients that won't affect weight loss on the HCG Diet. The Flavor drops are absolutely delicious on all phases of the diet when added to smoothies, beverages, entrees, and desserts, and are suitable to enjoy during the rapid weight loss of the *HCG Phase* (Phase 2 or P2) of the diet without slowing weight loss. I have added Flavor drops to some of the recipes in this book but they are optional. You can substitute a hint of vanilla, flavored Stevia, other calorie free/oil free Flavor drops, or spice mixes for the Flavor drops in the majority of the recipes, or feel free to omit them in any recipe. Flavor drops are available for purchase primarily from online retailers.

Flavors Used in This Book

(Optional)

Coconut

Butter or Popcorn

Cheesecake

Chocolate

Maple or French Toast

BRAGG'S LIQUID AMINOS

Bragg's liquid aminos is a calorie free soy sauce alternative that adds tremendous flavor to the recipes in this cookbook. If you find that it causes a slowing or stall in weight loss, or if you have concerns about the sodium content, feel free to reduce or eliminate it from the recipes. You may also adjust the amounts of Bragg's liquid aminos or any of the spices to your own personal taste. Bragg's liquid aminos can be purchased from most local health food stores, health oriented grocery stores, and online retailers.

APPLE CIDER VINEGAR

Apple cider vinegar is a delicious and healthful vinegar that is the recommended vinegar while on this diet and for the recipes in this cookbook. Apple cider vinegar is known to have tremendous health benefits. I suggest choosing a brand that is raw and organic. Apple cider vinegar can be found in most health food stores, grocery stores, and online retailers. Some other vinegars such as white wine, red wine, and rice vinegar may be substituted on occasion in the recipes in this cookbook, but please avoid any vinegars that have a high sugar content such as balsamic vinegar and vinegars with added sugars while on the *HCG Phase* (Phase 2 or P2) of the HCG Diet.

HCG DIET Tip *When you want something sweet, enjoy sugar free, diet friendly Flavor drops and flavored Stevia in your favorite beverage or make a fresh fruit dessert.*

The Well Stocked HCG Diet Kitchen

Cooking on the HCG Diet is a breeze when you have the right tools. Often, you may be the only member of your family on the diet and may have to prepare single serving, special HCG Diet meals for yourself. It's critical that the meals be separated and your meals prepared fat-free. In this section of the cookbook, I offer a few suggestions for properly stocking your kitchen with the right tools in preparation for single serving cooking on the HCG Diet.

Many of the items on the list you may already have in your kitchen and purchasing any or all items on this list is, of course, optional or easily substituted with a piece of cookware you already own. The focus of this section of the book is to help you prepare and adjust your cooking style to the smaller, single serving portions using properly sized cookware and dishes that will allow for cooking delicious, quick, easy meals while on the HCG Diet.

Bullet Blender

A bullet blender is perfect for preparing single serving HCG Diet meals, soups, and sauces. A bullet blender is also great for making smoothies, iced or blended coffee drinks, pureeing vegetables, and more. You may also choose to use a regular blender or food processor.

Small Sauté Pan

A small sauté pan is perfect for preparing single serving HCG Diet meals, particularly simple protein or egg dishes, heating leftovers, or cooking sauces.

Large Frying Pan

A large frying pan is very useful for cooking up multiple protein or vegetable servings or to accommodate bulky vegetable entrees using chard and cabbage.

Baking Sheet

A baking sheet is useful for creating **Melba Toast Croutons** or to use under smaller baking dishes to catch drippings. It is also perfect for single or multiple servings of chicken or fish baked dishes, or other items such as **Italian Chicken Nuggets**.

Small Baking Dishes, Brûlée Cups, Muffin Tins, and Mini Loaf Pans

I use brûlée cups often for things like baked desserts or single serving casseroles. You can find them at most stores that carry housewares or kitchen products. I like the 3.5 inch brûlée cups and find they are the perfect size for many of the baked entrees and desserts featured in the *HCG Diet Gourmet Cookbooks*.

Measuring Cups

In any well stocked kitchen you should have a measuring cup that measures up to 2 cups of liquid or other food items. It is helpful to have a complete set of measuring cups including 1/4 cup, 1/2 cup, 3/4 cup, and 1 cup.

Measuring Spoons

A must in any kitchen is a good set of measuring spoons: 1/8 teaspoon, 1/4 teaspoon, 1/2 teaspoon, 1 teaspoon, and 1 tablespoon. If you can't find one that measures 1/8 teaspoon then "guesstimate" half of a 1/4 teaspoon measuring spoon.

Set of Knives

A good set of knives is also essential to any well stocked kitchen. Smaller knives for mincing vegetables and herbs, slicing poultry, meats, and vegetables; and a steak knife for cutting your meat servings. I recommend a Chef's knife, a serrated medium size knife, a smaller mincing knife, a paring knife, and a set of steak knives.

Cutting Board

Another important item for any well stocked kitchen is a cutting board. I recommend choosing a cutting board made from an anti-bacterial material such as silicone or plastic as it is more sanitary than wood-based boards when preparing items such as meat, fish, or chicken.

Spatula, Flipper, Wooden Spoon, Soup Ladle, and Other Utensils

A good spatula and stirring spoons are useful for soups and scraping the pan for juices and sauces. I personally use a good silicon, heat resistant spatula which helps me get every last drop. A flat flipper spatula is good for flipping hamburgers and other patties, eggs, etc., and a quality soup ladle is a must for dishing out the delicious soups in this cookbook.

Colander

I use a colander to wash my fruits and vegetables (with a quality vegetable wash) as well as to strain any excess liquid from steaming vegetables.

Medium Sauce Pan (2 quarts)

This is the perfect size for making a hearty serving of HCG Diet Soup. It is large enough to accommodate the liquid as well as the bulky vegetables such as shredded cabbage.

Stock Pot

Useful for creating your own healthy broths, it is a useful addition to any well stocked kitchen, and can be used after the diet is over to make large servings of soups and chili.

HCG Diet Cooking Tips

One of the challenges on the HCG Diet is fat-free cooking. In this section of the book I will offer you a few of my favorite cooking tips for delicious and flavorful meals.

- Steam your vegetables in broth or water with Bragg's liquid aminos for added flavor.

- Cook multiple servings in a single pan and adjust the spices to your taste.

- Allow the pan to brown slightly while cooking meats or vegetables and then deglaze with water or broth to create a rich and flavorful sauce.

- Lightly brown beef before roasting or adding liquids.

- Cook sauces with lemon slices to add a tangy flavor.

- Adjust the spices, Bragg's liquid aminos, vinegar, etc. to your personal taste. Add Stevia for sweetness.

- To reduce the sodium content of many of the recipes, use less broth or Bragg's liquid aminos and add more water.

- Substitute any of the proteins, vegetables, or fruit in the recipes for even more variety with your meals.

- Prepare ingredients in advance. Chop vegetables and onions, and mince garlic in advance to reduce prep time when cooking. Keep sealed baggies of minced onions in the freezer to quickly and easily measure and use as you prepare your meals.

- To reduce the fat in ground beef, boil it in water and strain off the fat.

Cooking Terms

(All HCG Diet cooking methods are implemented without use of fat or oil.)

Poach: To cook an ingredient in a boiling or simmering liquid

Fry: To cook in a pan over direct heat

Sauté: To quickly fry in a hot pan

Stir Fry: To cut ingredients into small pieces and cook in a wok or frying pan over high heat

Bake: To cook using dry heat in an oven

Broil: To cook by high direct heat, over heat or in an oven under the heat

Braise: Meat is browned and then simmered over low heat until tender

Grill: To cook over a grate

Glaze: To coat with a glaze substance (verb), or the glaze substance itself (noun)

De-glaze: To add a liquid to a pan to create a sauce from the remaining cooking juices

Roast: To bake uncovered in an oven or on a spit

Whisk: To whip to a froth using a whisk or beating instrument

Blend: To combine ingredients together

Puree: Blend into a smooth consistency through a strainer or in a blender

Barbecue: To roast over an open flame or heat source. Often basted with a barbecue sauce.

Chop: To cut loosely into pieces

Mince: To cut or chop into very small pieces

Dice/Cube: To cut into cube-like pieces

Slice: To cut into slices/equal parts

Shred/Grate: To cut into small pieces using a grater

Julienne: To cut into long, thin strips

Measurements

1 Cup = 8 fluid ounces = 1/2 pint = 237 ml

1 Tablespoon = .5 ounces = 14.29 grams = .01417 kilos

1 Teaspoon = .333 tablespoons = .16666 ounces = 4.76 grams = .0047 kilos

Calorie: A unit for measuring heat, particularly the value of foods for producing heat and energy in the human body equivalent to the amount of heat required to raise the temperature of one kilogram of water one degree Celsius; used as a measurement of nutrition

Tbsp: Tablespoon

Tsp: Teaspoon

Dash: Less than 1/8 teaspoon

HCG
DIET
Tip

The secret to cooking flavorful meals for the HCG Diet is a good selection of spices. Avoid spices with MSG, starch or sugar.

Stabilization Secrets
(Phase 3 or P3)

When you reach the end of the *HCG Phase* (Phase 2 or P2), it is time to transition into the *Stabilization Phase* of the HCG Diet. This is a critical aspect of the diet and is the time when your body and weight stabilize and your new and faster metabolism kicks in. After your last dose of HCG, continue to observe the low calorie diet for 72 hours as the HCG leaves your system. You will then increase your calories to a normal amount and enjoy a wider variety of foods as long as they are free of starch and sugar.

The calories will vary per individual depending on height, weight, and activity level. For women it is usually approximately 1700-2500 calories per day and for men, 2200-2700 calories per day. It is important to start immediately eating normal calorie amounts and foods rather than continuing to diet and just doubling your portions. Many dieters feel apprehensive about eating more fat and calories and yet this is very important to stabilizing properly.

During the first few days and weeks on the *Stabilization Phase,* you can expect some wild swings as your weight fluctuates and then begins to stabilize. Do a Steak Day if you go two pounds over your LIW, as needed, and continue to eat normal calories and foods thereafter.

Stabilization Phase Foods

Proteins
Poultry

Chicken

Turkey

Duck

Meat

Beef

Buffalo

Venison

Lamb

Pork

Seafood

Fish (white, tuna, salmon, etc.)

Shrimp

Lobster and crab

Scallops

Other (caviar, other shellfish, etc.)

Eggs

Protein Powder

Egg white

Whey protein

Rice protein powder

Pea protein powder

Note: Choose high quality, naturally processed protein powders prepared without sugar or starch. Avoid protein powders prepared with soy or soy isolate.

Cheese

Cheddar

Gouda

Parmesan and Romano

Brie, feta and goats milk cheeses

Most other cheeses

Dairy Products (*Full fat dairy products only*)

Cream

Half and half

Greek yogurt

Nuts, Seeds, Nut Butters, and Nut Flours (*in small to moderate amounts*)

Almonds

Walnuts

Pistachios

Pecans

Macadamia nuts

Brazil nuts

Hazelnuts

Coconut flour

Almond flour

Peanut butter

Almond butter

Flax seeds

Chia seeds

Avoid: Cashews, chestnuts, sesame seeds, pumpkin seeds (pepitas) and sunflower seeds.

Note: Caution with nuts, seeds, and nut butters on the *Stabilization Phase*. Some dieters will not be able to tolerate them while others will be fine. Also be careful not to overindulge in them as a snack food.

H C G D I E T *Tip* — *On the Stabilization or Maintenance Phases, add powdered supplements to your smoothies or your green drink for extra nutrition.*

Vegetables

Leafy green vegetables (i.e. Lettuce, Kale, Spinach, Mustard and Collard greens, etc.)

Summer and yellow squashes

Zucchini

Cabbage

Brussel sprouts

Asparagus

Cauliflower

Rutabagas

Turnips

Eggplant

Mushrooms

Peppers and chilies (Bell pepper, chili peppers, ortega chilies, etc.)

Carrots (steamed due to the high sugar content found in raw carrots)

Tomatoes

All other non-starchy vegetables

Fruits

Apples

Pears

Pomegranates

Cherries

Peaches

Melons

Citrus fruits

Grapes

Kiwi

Most other fruits in moderation

Most fruits are fine on the *Stabilization Phase* (Phase 3 or P3). Enjoy them in moderation. You may want to avoid overindulging in some of the higher glycemic fruits such as pineapple, cherries, and oranges. Avoid bananas and all dried fruits due to the concentrated starch and sugar content. Still, you can enjoy most other fruits available to you on the *Stabilization Phase* without a problem.

Miscellaneous Foods and Specialty Ingredients

Vinegar (apple cider, red wine vinegar, white wine vinegar)

Natural, sugar free sweeteners (Stevia, Erythritol, Xylitol, food grade Vegetable glycerin)

Condiments, dressings, and sauces (as long as they are sugar and starch free)

Spices, fresh or dried

Teas, coffees, and other sugar free beverages

Defatted cocoa, powdered

Konjac flour (used as a thickener)

Kombucha drink

Note: Avoid Balsamic vinegar while on P3 due to sugar content

Fats and Oils

Olive oil

Coconut oil

Walnut oil

Hazelnut oil

Grapeseed oil

Sesame oil

Omega 3 oils (flax oil, fish oil, etc.)

Butter

Ghee

Note: Essential fatty acids are Omega 3s and Omega 6s. Both are necessary for good health but it is important to have a proper balance and have enough Omega 3s. Most people get too much Omega 6 and therefore, to create the proper balance, more Omega 3s are necessary.

Avoid processed fat in any form such as hydrogenated oils and trans fats. Eating oils in their most natural (first press, etc.) state is ideal. Extra virgin, first press olive oil and coconut oils are fabulous.

Coconut oil has gotten a bad rap in the past but it is now coming to light that it is incredibly healthful and may even help you lose weight. Foods like salmon, tuna and other fatty fish have high quality Omega 3 oils. Nuts such as walnuts and almonds are another good source of healthy fats, in addition to quality protein and antioxidants.

Foods to Enjoy Occasionally and in Moderation

Nuts, Seeds, Nut Butters, and Nut Flours

Alcoholic Beverages

Wine
Beer
Liquor (Gin, vodka, scotch, tequila, etc.)

Note: Avoid any sweet liqueurs or sugary mixers.

Foods to Avoid

Wheat bread, pasta, and other wheat products (including sprouted grain bread)

Rice and rice products

Corn and corn products

All other grains

Potatoes

Starchy vegetables such as winter squashes and parsnips

Nonfat and low fat dairy products (milk, cheese, yogurt)

Sugar, honey, agave, high fructose corn syrup, and other sugary sweeteners

Soda (regular and diet)

Artificial sweeteners, additives, chemicals, and processed foods

Balsamic vinegar (high sugar content)

Dried fruits

Excessive amounts of highly sugared fruits like cherries and pineapple

Bananas

Condiments, spices, and dressings that contain sugar

Shortening, margarine, and trans fat hydrogenated oils

Most soy products, especially processed soy products

Corn and food starch additives

Sweet liqueurs or sugary mixers

Cashews, chestnuts, pumpkin seeds (pepitas), safflower seeds, sunflower seeds, and sesame seeds

Stabilization Phase Sample Menus

Breakfast

Coffee or tea with cream or half and half, 3 egg omelet with vegetables and cheese

Coffee or tea with cream or half and half, 2 eggs, 2 pieces of breakfast meat, Greek yogurt with fruit

Lunch

Chef's salad with your choice of dressing

Grilled chicken breast topped with marinated or buttered mushrooms, sautéed herbed vegetables or green salad with dressing

Dinner

Grilled steak topped with blue cheese, grilled vegetables with olive oil and a green salad, and fresh berries with whipped cream

Herbed fish with white wine caper sauce, cauliflower risotto, and a mini cheesecake with raspberry sauce

Stabilization Phase Snacks

Cheese stick with fruit

Chopped raw vegetables with cheese or dip

Apple slices with cinnamon and walnuts

Almonds or 2 tablespoons peanut butter with apple slices

Slice of turkey, chicken, or beef with cheese rolled up or in a lettuce wrap

10-15 almonds or walnuts

Protein shake or smoothie (use a high quality sugar free whey, egg white, or rice protein mix) with ice, berries or other fruit

Fresh vegetable juice (serve with a splash of cayenne pepper sauce and black pepper)

1/2 cup of egg salad with raw vegetables or greens

Fruit salad

Raw veggie sticks with dip or a tablespoon of sugar free, natural peanut butter

HOT TIPS:

Avoid all sugar and starches in the *Stabilization Phase* (Phase 3 or P3). It is wise to check all ingredient lists for items you buy. Hidden sugars are often found in food items such as salad dressings, condiments, and processed food.

- Exercise caution when dining out as many restaurants add sugar to their sauces and marinades and this can cause weight gain during Phase 3.

- Choose high quality proteins and make sure you eat approximately half your weight in grams of protein every single day. Getting enough protein is essential during this phase because you have just come out of the *HCG Phase* where you are on the brink of protein deficiency.

Feel your best

The *Stabilization Phase* is a very important part of the HCG Diet. It is equally as important as the intensive weight loss experienced during the *HCG Phase*. The *Stabilization Phase* helps to lock in and stabilize your new and faster metabolism. It is wise to complete the full recommended three weeks on the *Stabilization Phase*. You should then be able to transition safely into the *Maintenance Phase* without weight gain. Continue monitoring your weight through all the Phases and notice which foods help you maintain your weight and feel your best.

- Consider the *Stabilization Phase* an opportunity to maximize your nutrition and choose healthy, nutrient-dense foods such as fruits and vegetables, especially if you have multiple rounds of HCG to do to reach your goal weight.

- Choose high quality fats and eat enough of them. Contrary to what many people believe, fat is actually good for you and essential for many bodily functions. You do not need to worry about fat during Phase 3 or even during the *Maintenance Phase* (Phase 4 or P4). In fact, it is actually better for you to eat full fat dairy, nuts, and oils than most nonfat diet foods.

- Many of the foods that are really wonderful for you, such as nuts, avocado, healthy oils, fatty fish, etc., are very high in fat. Train your brain away from choosing nonfat or diet food products and back into real, whole food eating habits that include reasonable amounts of fat both on Phase 3 and for the rest of your life.

- Take quality supplements to help build your nutrition back up after the restrictive *HCG Phase* and choose high quality, unprocessed foods, focusing on protein, fresh fruits and vegetables.

You will have more variety and choices on this phase with your meals and can even enjoy an alcoholic beverage on occasion.

- It is not advisable to continue to attempt more weight loss during this phase. The goal of the *Stabilization Phase* is to STABILIZE at your new weight and higher metabolism. Continuing to diet or lose more weight during this time may actually lower your metabolism and cause weight gain later.

- Feel free to exercise at a rate that is comfortable for you during this phase. You can take this opportunity to perform higher intensity workouts and focus on strength building, cardiovascular exercise and toning.

Maintenance Secrets

(Phase 4 or P4)

It is an incredible feeling when you finally reach your weight loss goal. For someone who has struggled with their weight, it is exhilarating to fit into those smaller jeans, breathe easier, and have more energy. Still, it can be daunting for dieters to consider the transition from the *Stabilization Phase* to the *Maintenance Phase* and wonder, "What foods can I eat?" and "How do I maintain my weight?"

As you move into the *Maintenance Phase,* or "The Rest of Your Life" you should notice that your metabolism is significantly improved and your weight is stabilized. You will be able to gradually re-introduce more carbohydrates and starches back into your diet and feel confident that you won't gain the weight back. This is the normal and healthy diet plan that you will enjoy for the rest of your life. The true secret of long-term maintenance following the HCG Diet is getting back to a whole food, more natural diet.

In my opinion, it is far more important during this phase to consider the kinds of foods you eat rather than the number of fat grams and calories. I want to encourage you to drop the "Diet" mentality and start living your life and choosing foods that energize you and keep you healthy. If you are just taking a break between rounds and still have more weight to lose, look at your time on the *Maintenance Phase* as a way to begin to adjust your lifestyle and break old habits from the past by making healthier food choices.

Maintenance Phase Foods

Proteins

Poultry
Chicken

Turkey

Duck

Other poultry

Meat
Beef

Buffalo

Venison

Lamb

Pork

Other meat

Seafood
Fish (white, tuna, salmon, etc.)

Shrimp

Lobster and crab

Scallops

Other seafood

Eggs

Protein Powder
Egg white

Whey protein

Rice protein powder

Pea protein powder

Note: Choose high quality, naturally processed protein powders prepared without sugar or starch. Avoid protein powders prepared with soy or soy isolate.

Cheese
Cheddar

Gouda

Parmesan and Romano Brie, Feta, and goats milk cheeses

Most other cheeses

Dairy Products
(Full fat dairy products only)
Cream

Half and half

Greek yogurt

Nuts, Seeds, Nut Butters, and Nut Flours
Almonds

Walnuts

Pistachios

Pecans

Macadamia nuts

Brazil nuts

Hazelnuts

Cashews

Pumpkin seeds (pepitas)

Coconut flour

Almond flour

Peanut butter

Almond butter

Flax seeds

Chia seeds

Sunflower seeds

Sesame seeds

(Nuts are a nutrient dense food and should be enjoyed in moderation as a healthy snack)

Vegetables
Leafy green vegetables (i.e. lettuce, kale, spinach, mustard and collar greens, etc.)

Summer and yellow squashes

Zucchini

Cabbage

Brussel sprouts

Asparagus

Cauliflower

Rutabagas

Turnips

Eggplant

Mushrooms

Peppers and chilies (bell pepper, chili peppers, ortega chilies, etc.)

Carrots (steamed or raw)

Tomatoes

Potatoes (starch)

Parsnips (starch)

Butternut and Acorn squashes (Starch)

All other vegetables

Fruits

Apples

Peaches

Nectarines

Grapes

Cherries

Strawberries and other berries such as blackberries, blueberries, raspberries

Melons

Oranges, lemons, limes, grapefruit, tangerines, and other citrus fruits

Pears

Pomegranates

Bananas (starch)

Pineapple

All other fruits including dried fruits, in moderation

Note: You are able to enjoy most fruits in moderation when you are on the *Maintenance Phase*. You may still wish to exercise caution in eating excessive amounts of super sweet fruits, starchy fruits such as bananas, or dried fruits (dehydrating concentrates the sugars, and commercially produced dried fruits often contain additives).

Miscellaneous Foods and Specialty Ingredients

Condiments, dressings, and sauces (low sugar and sugar free preferred)

Vinegars (apple cider, red wine, white wine, and including balsamic vinegar)

Natural sugar free sweeteners (Stevia, Erythritol, Xylitol, food grade Vegetable glycerine)

Raw honey and other natural sugars (in moderation)

Spices, fresh or dried

Konjac flour (used as a thickener)

Teas, coffee, defatted cocoa, and other sugar free beverages

Dark chocolate

Kefir (unsweetened)

Kombucha drink

Fats and Oils

Olive oil

Coconut oil

Walnut oil

Hazelnut oil

Grapeseed oil

Sesame oil

Omega 3 oils (flax oil, fish oil, etc.)

Butter

Ghee

Cream

Nut and seed oils like walnut, hazelnut, grapeseed, and sesame

Starches and Grains

Sprouted grain bread

Rice

Oatmeal

Quinoa

Beans and legumes

Lentils

Starchy squashes (i.e. winter squash, acorn, and butternut squash)

Potatoes and sweet potatoes

Parsnips

Carrots

Plantains

Corn

Foods to Enjoy Occasionally and in Moderation

Starches and grains (3 servings or less per day)

Wheat bread, pasta, and other starches containing gluten

Honey and other natural sugars

Dried fruits

Alcoholic beverages and sweet liqueurs

Foods to Avoid

Overly processed food

Artificial sweeteners (found in many processed foods and diet sodas/drinks)

Artificial flavors, colors, and chemical food additives

H C G
D I E T
Tip

On the Stabilization and Maintenance Phases, eat small meals, snacks, and calories throughout the day to give you extra energy and keep your metabolism up.

MSG (monosodium glutamate, a chemical flavor enhancer)

Aspartame, Sucralose, Saccharine, Acesulfame K, and other chemical sweeteners

Excessive white/processed sugar

Excessive white bread, pasta, or processed grain products

Trans fats and hydrogenated oils

High fructose corn syrup (found in most processed food, soda, and drinks)

Excessive fructose (as found in fruits and fruit juices)

Most soy products, especially processed soy products and isolate

Maintenance Phase Sample Menus

Breakfast

Oatmeal topped with fruit, cream, and Stevia with 2 scrambled eggs

2 eggs or veggie omelet with cheese, fruit, and buttered sprouted grain toast

Lunch

Stir fried vegetables with chicken or shrimp over brown rice

Sprouted grain sandwich with cheese, lettuce or roasted veggies, and meat of choice

Dinner

Steak topped with onions and blue cheese with buttered vegetables, herbed potatoes, and Blackberry Panna Cotta

Baked Chicken Parmesan with grilled roasted vegetables, mushroom risotto and fresh fruit trifle

Maintenance Snacks

Toast with peanut butter or cottage cheese and fresh tomatoes

Deviled eggs and celery sticks

A cup of quinoa salad with vegetables and chicken

A mini turkey, cheese, and veggie roll-up in 1/4 of a sprouted grain tortilla

A kefir smoothie with protein powder and fresh fruit

Trail mix/nuts

Fruit and walnuts with honey sweetened Greek yogurt

> *Cheers* Congratulations to you on your HCG Diet success and your transition to Maintenance! There are very few restrictions on the *Maintenance Phase* as far as the kinds of foods you can eat, and you can have most foods in moderation. You will find that there are healthy versions of just about any food you enjoy. It's a wonderful feeling to ditch the "diet food" in your cupboard and just eat a real, home cooked meal. As you move forward into the future, I suggest that you enjoy a wide variety of nutritious whole foods and observe a healthy lifestyle. Enjoy your life to the fullest!

HOT TIPS:

- Choose high fiber, whole foods as unprocessed as possible whenever you can. Getting away from processed food loaded with additives, chemicals, and sugar is critical for successfully maintaining your weight after the HCG Diet is over.

- Enjoy nutrient dense foods that are rich in vitamins and minerals such as fruits and vegetables. You will find that the more nutrients your body is receiving from your food, the less you will crave sugar, processed carbohydrates, and junk food. The body often signals you to eat larger quantities of food because it is demanding more nutrients from the foods you are eating. When you are eating devitalized, overly processed food, your body may be crying out for nutrients and triggering excessive hunger and cravings.

- Minimize or eliminate sugar in your diet, particularly processed varieties like high fructose corn syrup and white refined sugar. You will find that just about any food can be enjoyed in moderation on the *Maintenance Phase* but the evidence is compelling that sugar has an addictive quality, in addition to contributing to diabetes and other health issues.

- Enjoy eating small meals throughout the day and plenty of snacks. You should never allow yourself to get too hungry. I carry a bag of nuts, some cheese sticks, or fruit with me at all times. In fact, it seems I'm always eating. It's important to eat plenty of calories and eat the right kind of foods often.

- Limit your daily grain and starchy vegetable servings to 3 or less per day.

- Combine high carbohydrate, grain, starch, or sweet foods with a serving of fat or protein to decrease the glycemic load and balance the impact of these foods on blood sugar.

- When choosing foods to enjoy as part of the *Maintenance Phase* of the HCG Diet, choose starches and carbohydrates in their most natural form containing all the fiber, nutrients, vitamins, and minerals.

Health and Wellness Secrets

The primary goal of the HCG Diet is to stabilize and maintain weight for life. In this section, I want to address some general principles for good health that will help you maintain your weight long after the HCG Diet is over. When you begin this journey of weight loss transformation with the HCG Diet you will discover many things about yourself. You begin to look at the food you eat and your body differently and begin to shift your habits and lifestyle to make positive changes. Many of the following health ideas and concepts can greatly assist with the process of losing weight and keeping it off during and after the Program. Health and Wellness Secrets applies to your everyday life and expresses a word or two about various health philosophies that will help guide you to lasting success. They may seem like common sense and are certainly not new. Whether you try one or all of them, I hope that you find them informative and helpful for you.

Organic

Organic is becoming even more and more important. Our food supply contains many toxins, pesticides, hormones, and other processing ingredients that have detrimental effects on our health. In my opinion, it is animal products that can be the most dangerous — eggs, milk and dairy products, meat and poultry products, farmed fish, and seafood.

Choosing organic fruits and vegetables is ideal as it is believed that they contain higher levels of nutrition. If it is impossible or difficult to get organic fruits and vegetables, make sure you use a good vegetable wash to ensure that you get the surface pesticides off the food. Some of the worst offenders that are heavily sprayed with toxic chemicals are berries, oranges, and coffee.

Detoxification

Detoxifying the body is a well known practice that can improve the way your body functions and the way you feel. Some detox regimens to consider are colon cleansing, liver cleansing, candida cleanses, dry brushing, infrared saunas, and epsom salt baths. Detoxing can sometimes make you feel worse before you get better due to the release of toxins into the body. Drinking lots of water during the process can assist in the removal of those toxins and keep you hydrated. It is wise to be monitored by a health professional, particularly if you are performing an aggressive detox procedure or have health issues.

Nutrition

PROTEIN

Choosing the right kinds of foods for health and wellness can help you maintain your new weight for life following the HCG Diet. Eating enough protein is essential, since protein is the building block for all body tissues and systems. I recommend eating approximately half your body weight in grams of high quality protein per day (for example, if you weigh 130 pounds, I recommend eating approximately 65 grams of high quality protein per day).

FAT

Contrary to popular opinion, fat is a really important part of your diet. You need the Omega 3 oils found in fish and flax seed oil for many of the body's basic functions.

The low-fat diet craze as represented in the supermarket with whole product lines of fat-free and low-fat food have actually contributed to weight gain in society.

Fat, along with protein and fiber, actually helps to slow down the release of sugars and carbohydrates into the bloodstream, which contribute to insulin resistance and diabetes. Fat also helps you feel sated after a meal so you don't feel hungry or overeat. Choosing full fat dairy, taking

supplements, eating fatty fish like salmon and tuna, and eating plenty of healthy oils like coconut and olive is a wonderful way to get those Omega 3 fatty acids on a regular basis.

CARBOHYDRATES

Many people have an absolute phobia about eating carbohydrates and while it is true that excessive carbohydrates (particularly the white processed ones) can lead to weight gain, not all carbohydrates are created equal. As a general rule, most of your carbs should come from fresh fruits and vegetables, but it is also fine to enjoy some grain servings or starchy vegetables when on the *Maintenance Phase*. I recommend choosing high fiber, nutrient dense carbohydrates whenever possible, and limit your servings to 2-3 grain servings per day. Some people have a sensitivity to wheat products so choosing alternative grains like quinoa, sprouted grain, rice, and corn are generally better choices than a wheat muffin or a morning bowl of cereal.

SUPPLEMENTS

Supplements can be a healthy addition to your new lifestyle. The basic daily supplements I take personally are:

A whole food vitamin and/or a quality green drink 1-2 times daily

Fish, flax, or other healthy oil containing Omega 3 fatty acids

Digestive enzymes taken with meals

Probiotics

Trace minerals

Magnesium taken as a supplement or applied topically

Important things to consider when choosing supplements are the quality and source (choose a trusted manufacturer), and making sure to take them in a safe amount that can be utilized well by your body. Check with your healthcare professional for specialized nutritional and health recommendations. Some nutritional supplements may interfere with prescription medications.

While it is not recommended to take most supplements while on the *HCG Phase*, taking high quality supplements regularly is a way to ensure that you are receiving adequate nutrition throughout the other phases and for life.

Processed Foods and Additives

One of the secrets to maintaining weight following the HCG Diet is to observe a whole food, healthy, unprocessed, high fiber diet, rich in fruits and vegetables.

Many convenience and processed foods contain additives that are very unhealthy and can contribute to weight gain and poor health. There are far too many additives to mention them all by name in this book but, in general, I recommend learning to read food labels and eliminating food containing chemical sounding names.

Some of the worst offenders in the modern diet are artificial sweeteners like aspartame and sucralose, nitrites/nitrates, MSG, high fructose corn syrup, trans fats, and artificial preservatives.

Stress

Many healthcare professionals now recognize that managing stress levels is very important for good health. Some stress is positive in that it is motivating and energizing, but chronic negative stress often caused by challenging and stressful situations in life can cause physical and emotional ailments such as headaches, depression, anxiety, decreased adrenal function, and insomnia. Finding ways to decrease stress will improve your mental and emotional health and quality of life.

Guidelines for Success

A few ways to decrease your stress level are to take a walk or do some form of exercise regularly, get out in nature, listen to relaxing music, spend some quiet time in meditation, and have a positive outlook on life. Everybody has stress in their life, whether good or bad, and when we deal with whatever challenges we face in a positive manner we have a greater ability to create a healthier and happier life.

Attitude

Optimism and a positive attitude can make all the difference in your quality of life, stress level, and health. Let go of negative thoughts and emotions. Forgive people who have hurt you and choose to see the best in every situation. People who are able to see the silver lining, laugh as often as they can, and choose positivity have found one of the keys to happiness and success in life.

Restaurants

Restaurant dining on the HCG Diet can be a challenge. On the *HCG Phase* (P2 or Phase 2), the food choices, restrictions of oils, and cooking methods are so limited that restaurant dining can make it difficult to stay true to the diet. On the *Stabilization Phase* (P3 or Phase 3) more variety and food choices open up and the challenge becomes choosing entrees that

observe the strict "no starch/no sugar" requirements of the diet. It is difficult, but not impossible, to enjoy a meal out while on the HCG Diet. It does take preparation and care to ensure success and avoid weight gain the following day.

DINING OUT ON THE HCG PHASE

Order a salad, plate of raw spinach, or sliced tomatoes with a simply prepared, oil free protein like chicken breast.

Dress up restaurant meals with fresh lemon juice and herbs, cayenne pepper sauce, or fresh black pepper.

Clarify your diet needs with the chef or your server to ensure that your meal will be prepared without oil or sugar.

Enjoy a cup of coffee or hot green or herbal tea instead of dessert.

DINING OUT ON THE STABILIZATION PHASE

Skip the bread.

Ask your server about entrees that are prepared without sugar.

Order all sauces and dressings on the side. Many sauces contain sugar. You will have greater success and control avoiding sweet sauces when they are ordered on the side.

Ask for extra vegetables instead of starchy side dishes.

Order fresh fruit instead of sugary desserts.

DINING OUT ON THE MAINTENANCE PHASE
(i.e. for the rest of your life)

Choose healthy entrees and meals that have protein as the primary ingredient.

Enjoy extra vegetables and salads over starchy side dishes.

Limit grain and starch servings to one for that meal.

Order sauces on the side and minimize foods that contain sugar.

Limit your bread intake to one piece and eat it with a protein, olive oil, or butter.

If you choose to have dessert, share it or just have a few bites.

Stop eating when you are full and take the leftovers home.

RESTAURANT TIPS FOR ALL PHASES

Avoid fast food and most chain restaurants.

Carry packets of Stevia with you to add to hot and cold beverages.

Share a meal. Many restaurant portions contain 3 or more servings and sharing a meal is generally more than enough food to satisfy you. If you don't wish to share, ask the waiter to box up half of your meal before it is served so you can take it home and aren't tempted to overeat.

Chew your food well and savor each bite.

Focus on friends and family, the experience, and the fun of dining out rather than the food itself.

Exercise

Exercise is a wonderful and healthy habit to incorporate into your life. During the *HCG Phase* and while eating a restricted calorie diet, it is not recommended to exercise heavily and may even stall weight loss. According to Dr. Simeons, the HCG is metabolizing fat at a rapid rate and you are on such a low calorie diet that aggressive exercise during this time could cause you to feel excessively hungry or even weak. It could also cause possible stalls due to mild and temporary water retention during the *HCG Phase*. Exercises that are acceptable during the *HCG Phase* are walking, stretching, rebounding, light yoga stretching, and swimming. During the other phases and for life, work out and exercise at a level that is comfortable for your age and health. Cardiovascular exercise, weight training and toning, intensive exercise classes, jogging, etc., are great during other phases of the diet and have tremendous health benefits for your heart, circulation, strength, and overall fitness. When beginning any exercise program, check with your doctor first and begin slowly, at a pace that is appropriate for your health, age, and activity level.

Cheating and Hunger

I wanted to address the issue of cheating on the HCG Diet because so many dieters have struggled with this issue and it is vitally important to remain true to the Diet to achieve the best results.

I know how tempting it can be to cheat, especially on the low calorie *HCG Phase*, but cheating is simply not an option on this diet. You absolutely cannot and should not cheat. The fact is, one single bite of something other than the allowable foods on the *HCG Phase* of the diet can result in significant weight gain and up to 3 days or more of stalled weight loss.

The other phase that dieters sometimes struggle with the issue of cheating is the *Stabilization Phase*. Because of the rich variety of foods allowed on the *Stabilization Phase* it is easy to underestimate its importance. The *Stabilization Phase* is the time when your weight loss stabilizes at a new level. It is very important to observe the rule of avoiding all starch and sugar during this time and maintaining your weight within the 2 pound range around your LIW. If you find that you are tempted to cheat and eat foods like bread or sugar, I recommend that you focus again on the end result and just don't do it.

Choices On the *Maintenance Phase* there really is no cheating and there should be no hunger because you are eating plenty of food and calories. Remember, the goal is to get away from "dieting" altogether once the diet is over. Therefore, your food choices simply become a matter of common sense and you should never feel like you must deny yourself, but rather eat in a way that feels good to your body and gives you energy.

HOT TIPS:

To help you avoid the disheartening and unnecessary weight gain and struggle, I'm including a few tips on how to avoid cheating on the HCG Diet:

- If you find yourself tempted, remind yourself that your time on the restricted calorie *HCG Phase* of the HCG Diet is only 3-6 weeks and that you will return to normal calories and a healthy diet very soon. Focus on delayed gratification right now and how wonderful you will look and feel when you are at your goal weight.

- To deal with hunger and avoid cheating, always have a snack ready (fruit, celery sticks, protein, etc.). You can save your second fruit serving for the evening if you tend to get cravings late at night. If you have a sweet tooth, you can make one of the desserts from this cookbook and that alone can often satisfy you enough to avoid cheating.

- Drink extra water. Add a squeeze of lemon and a little Stevia to your water if you are craving sweets. The water will help fill you up and also help flush toxins from your system as you lose weight.

- Eat extra vegetables for that meal or make warm and filling soup.

- Have a cup of any of the recommended teas.

- Ask yourself if you are actually hungry. Sometimes, the feeling interpreted as "hunger" is actually just missing some of the foods you used to eat. It can also be a sign of dehydration that can be easily remedied by drinking extra water.

- To resist cheating, journal all the reasons why you want to lose the weight. Is it for your family? Your kids? Your health? Looking good and wearing beautiful clothes? Remembering why you chose to lose the weight in the first place and knowing the consequences if you cheat can help you stay on track with your weight loss program.

- Think about the end result. Visualize yourself at your goal weight. See yourself being more active, playing with your kids, and buying that new bikini. Make these your goals and a reason not to cheat. Take a walk. A quick walk around the block and some fresh air and sunshine can help you clear your head and get your mind off food and the temptation of cheating.

- Get your family and friends on board. Many times people cheat because they are confronted with temptation. Ask your family and friends not to offer you foods that tempt you to cheat and to support you during your time on the HCG Diet.

- Join a support group. Having people around who understand what you are going through with the HCG Diet is very important. If you are having a bad day and are tempted to cheat, you can turn to them for helpful advice and emotional support.

Most of all, remember this is a temporary diet and the results are long lasting. You will not be on the *HCG Phase* of the HCG Diet forever. You will eat normal, healthy, food and calories again. Focus on the delayed gratification right now and think about how healthy and attractive you will be when you reach your goal weight and stick with the plan. It will be worth it.

Mindset

As you begin this process of losing weight with the HCG Diet, it is important to begin to reshape your thoughts and feelings about your body and the foods you choose to eat. So many of us who have struggled with our weight have suffered from body issues and insecurities as a result of, and that perpetuate, the condition of being overweight.

Having the right mindset as you begin this journey is really important. Getting comfortable and clear about your goals and changing feelings about food and your body can be a critical element to your success through all the phases and especially maintaining your weight when the diet is over.

It takes the drive, the desire, new choices, and commitment to keep the weight off for good.

The HCG Phase Mindset

Focus on the end result and your goal. Remember that this is unlike any diet you've ever done before and the results are long lasting. Focus on delayed gratification rather than missing certain foods or old eating habits.

Measure yourself regularly and weigh yourself daily. Think about the lost inches and the looseness of your clothing and stay positive about the changes going on within your body.

Imagine buying smaller and more flattering clothes, wearing a bikini again, the activities and fun you will have when you are slimmer and feel more attractive. Get comfortable with the idea of being slim and begin to feel beautiful in your body no matter what your weight is right now.

The Stabilization Phase Mindset

Continue focusing on the end result and how great it will feel to be at your goal weight. Start shifting your feelings about food. Start thinking of food as a part of your life that nourishes, gives energy to your body, and is a source of pleasure, but isn't the central focus.

Stick to the allowed foods on this phase and recommit to the importance of stabilizing your weight and your metabolism.

Discover fun things other than food to reward yourself with, like seeing a movie, spending time with friends and family, or getting a massage.

Think about ways to reduce your stress, like exercise, meditation, dancing, doing something fun, listening to music, or other relaxing activities.

If you have more weight to lose, when you return to the *HCG Phase*, be proud and know that you are one step closer to your ultimate weight loss goal.

The Maintenance Phase Mindset

Gradually adjust your lifestyle, choices, and feelings about food and your body to reflect the positive new changes you now see in the mirror.

Continue the positive habits you've developed during the course of this diet and love your body, have some fun, and stay optimistic. Look at what you've accomplished and feel the sense of pride that comes from reaching your goal.

Remember your emotional triggers and the reasons why you are committed to maintaining your weight. It is helpful to continue to journal your food choices and feelings.

Take it easy on yourself. Don't beat yourself up if you gain a pound or eat something you feel you shouldn't. Most foods can be enjoyed in moderation while maintaining after the HCG Diet.

Drop the "diet" mindset once and for all. Start eating and enjoying real, healthy, whole food in normal amounts without obsessing over fat and calories. In reality, maintaining weight loss after the HCG Diet is more about the kinds of foods you choose to eat than fat grams and counting calories.

Maintaining after the HCG Diet is about making positive choices and developing a new way of looking at food and your body. It's about enjoying life and being free from the excess weight that has previously held you back from the life and body that you want. I wish you all the best as you move through the phases of the HCG Diet and lose the weight once and for all. I'm here to support you and cheer you on as you transform and adjust your mind to the incredible changes taking place in your body.

Mindset Exercises

- Prepare, plan, and write down your weight loss goals.

- Write down all the reasons why you want to lose the weight and read it to yourself regularly.

- Keep a journal to track your progress and keep you motivated throughout the weight loss process.

- Evaluate your thoughts and belief systems and analyze what experiences and feelings in your life have contributed to unhealthy or emotional eating patterns, food cravings, and negative behaviors.

- Gather support from your family or join a support group and prepare yourself mentally for the changes ahead as you begin the diet.

Dressings, Sauces and Marinades

Ranch Vinaigrette

Strawberry Dipping Sauce

Sweet Onion Vinaigrette

Sage Citrus Sauce/Dressing/Marinade

Cilantro Lemon Sauce/Dressing

Salsa Sauce

Teriyaki Sauce

Sweet Lemon Ginger Sauce/Dressing

Sweet and Sour Sauce

Ranch Vinaigrette

Ingredients
1/2 cup broth (choose a broth appropriate for the protein for that meal)
1 tablespoon apple cider vinegar
1 teaspoon lemon juice
1 teaspoon onion, minced
1/2 clove garlic, crushed and minced
1/4 teaspoon chives, fresh or dried (optional)
1/4 teaspoon minced parsley, fresh or dried (optional)
1/8 teaspoon garlic powder
1/8 teaspoon onion powder
1/8 teaspoon paprika
1/8 teaspoon dill
Pinch of Stevia
Salt and pepper to taste

Makes 1 serving

.05 gram protein

0 grams fat

5 calories

PHASE 3
MODIFICATIONS: Chill
reduced broth and
spice, omit apple cider
vinegar, and stir in 2
tablespoons of sour
cream or Greek yogurt
to make a delicious dip.

▶ Combine spices with broth and bring to a boil. Reduce heat and simmer for approximately 5 minutes until liquid is reduced by half. Allow to cool or chill for a cold dressing. Add apple cider vinegar and serve over salad greens.

Strawberry Dipping Sauce

Ingredients
3 strawberries
1 tablespoon lemon juice
Pinch of cayenne pepper to taste
Stevia to taste

Makes 1 serving
(1 fruit)

0 protein

0 grams fat

16 calories

▶ Puree strawberries with spices. Warm slightly to thicken and combine flavors. Serve warm or chilled. Add a teaspoon of apple cider vinegar to make a tangy dressing.

Serving Suggestion: Use as a dipping sauce for **Italian Chicken Nuggets**, **Chicken Strips**, or **Coconut Shrimp**.

Variation: Freeze pureed strawberry mixture for a sweet dessert.

Sweet Onion Vinaigrette

Ingredients
3 tablespoons broth
1-2 teaspoons apple cider vinegar or broth
1/4 teaspoon Bragg's liquid aminos
2 tablespoons onion, minced
Stevia to taste
Salt and pepper to taste

Makes 1 serving
0 grams protein
0 grams fat
16 calories

▶ Sauté onions and garlic in small saucepan. Add broth and additional spices and cook for approximately 3 minutes, stirring frequently. Remove from heat and stir in apple cider vinegar and Stevia to taste. Enjoy as a salad dressing.

Variations: Substitute 2 cloves garlic, crushed and minced, in place of the onion. Omit Stevia for a savory dressing.

Sage Citrus Sauce/Dressing/Marinade

Ingredients
3 orange segments, peeled (eat the rest of the orange to complete a
   fruit serving)
1/4 cup water
1 tablespoon lemon juice
5 fresh sage leaves, minced (substitute 1/4 teaspoon powdered)
1 tablespoon onion, minced
Pinch of lemon zest
Stevia to taste

Makes 1 serving (1 fruit)
0 protein
0 grams fat
17 calories

▶ Puree ingredients together. Simmer on low heat until sauce thickens.
Add 1 teaspoon apple cider vinegar to make a dressing/marinade.

Variations: Add a little cayenne pepper or vanilla.

Cilantro Lemon Sauce/Dressing

Ingredients
1/4 cup water (substitute chicken broth
   if paired with chicken for that meal)
3 slices lemon with rind
1 clove garlic, crushed and minced
6 fresh cilantro leaves, minced
Pinch of Stevia to taste (optional)
Salt and pepper to taste

Makes 1 serving
0 protein
0 grams fat
<.5 calories

▶ Sauté lemon slices in chicken broth, water, and spices. Simmer on low heat for about five minutes until sauce thickens. Remove rind and add water until desired consistency is reached.

Salsa Sauce

Ingredients
1 cup tomatoes, chopped
1/4 cup apple cider vinegar
1 teaspoon lemon juice
1 clove garlic, crushed and minced
1 tablespoon cilantro, chopped
1 tablespoon onion, minced
1/4 teaspoon oregano
Pinch cayenne pepper to taste
Salt and pepper to taste

Makes 1 serving
(1 vegetable)
3 grams protein
0 grams fat
37 calories

▶ Puree ingredients together in blender until smooth (or pulse for a chunkier texture). Serve chilled or warm the sauce for 1-3 minutes on low heat. Enjoy over your choice of protein.

HCG DIET Tip
Eat the rest of your fruit or vegetable serving if you use some of them in a sauce. Have some fresh tomato slices, strawberries, or oranges on the side to complete a full serving for that meal.

Teriyaki Sauce

Ingredients
1/2 cup beef or chicken broth (use a broth compatible with
  the protein for that meal)
3 tablespoons Bragg's liquid aminos
3 tablespoons lemon juice
2 tablespoons apple cider vinegar
Orange juice from 4 segments
1 tablespoon onion, minced
1 teaspoon garlic powder
1 teaspoon onion powder
2 cloves garlic, minced
1/2 teaspoon ginger, powdered or fresh grated
Pinch of lemon zest
Stevia to taste

Makes 1 serving
(1 fruit)

.5 grams protein

0 grams fat

18 calories

Combine all ingredients in a small saucepan and bring to a boil.
Reduce heat and simmer for 20 minutes or until liquid is reduced.
The longer you simmer, the richer the flavors. As the liquid reduces,
deglaze the pan to desired consistency with a little water to intensify the
flavors. Enjoy as a glaze or sauce with chicken, beef, or tossed into a salad.

Sweet Lemon Ginger Sauce/Dressing

Ingredients
1/2 cup water
2 lemon slices with rind
1 teaspoon fresh ginger, grated (substitute 1/4 teaspoon powdered)
Pinch of black pepper or cayenne pepper (optional)
Stevia to taste
Salt and pepper to taste

Makes 1 serving

0 protein

0 grams fat

<.5 calories

Sauté lemon slices in water with spices until liquid is reduced and sauce
is slightly thickened. Remove lemon rind and serve. To make dressing,
allow the sauce to cool and add 1 tablespoon apple cider vinegar. Serve as
a topping for protein or mixed into cabbage, spinach or salad greens.

Sweet and Sour Sauce

Ingredients

3/4 cup water

3 orange segments (eat the rest of the orange at that meal
   to complete a fruit serving)

3 lemon segments

2 teaspoons Bragg's liquid aminos

1 tablespoon apple cider vinegar

1 tablespoon hot sauce

1 tablespoon onion, minced

1/2 teaspoon fresh ginger

1/8 teaspoon garlic powder

1/8 teaspoon onion powder

Pinch of lemon and orange zest

Cayenne pepper or red pepper flakes to taste

Stevia to taste

Salt and pepper to taste

Makes 1 serving (1 fruit)
2 grams protein
0 grams fat
22 calories

Lightly crush or puree orange and lemon slices, spices, and liquid
ingredients, and bring to a boil in small saucepan. Reduce heat
and simmer for approximately 7-10 minutes until sauce is slightly
thickened. Add water as needed. Serve warm with your protein for
that meal or chill and stir into salads or as a dipping sauce.

Snacks and Appetizers

Cheese and Chive Appetizer

Spicy Onion Petals

Melba Toast Crumbs/Croutons

French Onion Dip

Shrimp on Toast

Hot Pickled Vegetables

Cheese and Chive Appetizer

Ingredients
100 grams nonfat cottage cheese
1 Melba toast
2 tablespoons chives, fresh or dried (or substitute minced green onion)
1/8 teaspoon garlic powder
Pinch of paprika
Salt and pepper to taste

Makes 1 serving
(1 protein, 1 Melba toast

18 grams protein
.5 grams fat
106 calories

> Mix cheese with spices and chives. Top with sprinkle of paprika or fresh ground black pepper and serve with Melba toast.

Serving Suggestion: Puree for a creamy dip. Serve with fresh sliced tomatoes or celery sticks.

Spicy Onion Petals

Ingredients
1/2 onion, cut into petals
1 serving **Melba Toast Crumbs**
1 tablespoon lemon juice
1/8 teaspoon parsley (optional)
1/8 teaspoon garlic powder
Pinch of paprika
Pinch of cayenne pepper
Salt and pepper to taste

Makes 1 serving
(1 vegetable, 1 Melba toast)

1 gram protein
0 grams fat
47 calories

> Marinate onion in liquid. Coat with **Melba Toast Crumbs** and bake at 400 degrees for approximately 10 minutes.

Serving Suggestion: Enjoy with a dipping sauce, cheese dip, or dressing.

Melba Toast Crumbs/Croutons

Ingredients
1 Melba toast
Lemon juice
Your choice of spices or herb mixes (e.g. **Savory Herb** and **Sweet Cinnamon** below)
Salt (optional)

Makes 1 serving
(1 Melba toast)
.5 gram protein
0 grams fat
22 calories

 Place Melba toast in small plastic bag or folded in plastic wrap. Crush Melba toast into powder with a rolling pin or flat object.

Serving Suggestion: Mix with your favorite spices and use as a topping for baked dishes or desserts.

Savory Herb
Ingredients
Pinch of paprika
Pinch of thyme
Pinch of garlic powder
Pinch of onion powder
Pinch of cayenne pepper
Salt and pepper to taste

Sweet Cinnamon
Ingredients
1/8 teaspoon cinnamon or to taste
Stevia to taste

Sprinkle the Melba toast with lemon juice and spices and bake for 5 minutes in a 400 degree oven or dust dry pieces with spices.

French Onion Dip

Ingredients
100 grams nonfat cottage cheese
1 tablespoon onion, minced
1 clove garlic, crushed and minced
1/8 teaspoon onion powder
1/8 teaspoon garlic powder
Cayenne pepper to taste
Pinch of Stevia

Makes 1 serving
(1 protein, 1 vegetable)
18 grams protein
.5 gram fat
89 calories

▶ Puree cottage cheese with spices. Serve with celery sticks or other allowed vegetable or serve atop a green salad.

Shrimp on Toast

Ingredients
2 cooked shrimp, peeled
2 slices cucumber
1 Melba toast
1/2 teaspoon cayenne pepper sauce
1/4 teaspoon Bragg's liquid aminos
Pinch of minced green onion
Salt and pepper to taste

Makes 1 serving
(1 protein, 1 vegetable, 1 Melba toast)
Complete a full protein and vegetable serving by eating a full 100 grams of shrimp and additional cucumber with the meal.
3.5 grams protein
.5 gram fat
35 calories

PHASE 3 MODIFICATIONS: Top cucumber with a thin layer of cream cheese and omit the Melba toast.

▶ Sauté shrimp in pepper sauce and aminos until cooked. Break Melba toast into two pieces and top with cucumber slice and shrimp. Top with green onion and serve.

Hot Pickled Vegetables

Ingredients
1 cup radishes, cabbage or celery, diced
1/2 cup apple cider vinegar
1 ring of onion, cut into strips
1 clove garlic, crushed and minced
1/2 teaspoon salt
1/4 teaspoon garlic powder
Pinch of cayenne pepper/red pepper flakes

▶ Loosely dice or chop vegetables and place in a small container or jar. Sprinkle liberally with salt and spices. Cover with apple cider vinegar, and marinate 24-48 hours in the refrigerator.

Serving Suggestion: Add to **Egg Salad** or serve as a side dish or snack.

Makes 1 serving
(1 vegetable)

1 gram protein

0 grams fat

20 calories

PHASE 3
MODIFICATIONS: Add additional vegetables such as slices of carrots, onion, bell pepper, etc.

Soups

Southwest Tomato Soup

Curried Chicken and Fennel Soup

HCG Diet Broth (Chicken, Beef, and
   Vegetable)

Reuben Soup

Rosemary Chicken Soup

Herbed Asparagus Soup

Curried Beef Soup

Gingered Fennel Soup

Savory Beef and Asparagus Soup

Hot and Sour Egg Drop Soup

Chilled Cucumber Soup

Italian Wedding Soup

Gingered Shrimp Soup

Tomato Meatball Soup

Beef and Spinach Stew

HCG Diet Soup

Southwest Tomato Soup

Ingredients

1 1/2 cups tomatoes, chopped
1 cup water (substitute allowed broth if desired)
1 tablespoon lemon juice
1 teaspoon Bragg's liquid aminos
2 cloves garlic, crushed and minced
1-2 tablespoons fresh cilantro
1 tablespoon onion, minced
1 teaspoon cumin
1/2 teaspoon garlic powder
1/2 teaspoon oregano
Cayenne pepper to taste
Salt and pepper to taste

Makes 1 serving
(1 vegetable)
4 grams protein
0 grams fat
55 calories

> Combine tomatoes, liquid ingredients and spices, and puree.
> Pour into a saucepan and simmer on low heat for 15-20 minutes,
> stirring occasionally. Serve topped with additional cilantro if desired.

Curried Chicken and Fennel Soup

Ingredients

100 grams chicken breast, cubed
1 1/2 cups fennel bulb, diced
1 1/2 cups water
1 cup chicken broth
1 tablespoon Bragg's liquid aminos
1 tablespoon chopped green onion
1 teaspoon curry powder
1/8 teaspoon fresh ginger, grated
Pinch of red pepper flakes
Stevia to taste

Makes 1 serving
(1 protein, 1 vegetable)
27 grams protein
2 grams fat
180 calories

> Bring water, broth, chicken, fennel and spices to a boil. Reduce heat
> and simmer for 20-25 minutes until fennel is tender and chicken is
> cooked.

Variations: Enjoy with a dash of cinnamon and a little Stevia.

HCG Diet Broth

All broths should be made only with meat (no bones).
Use only allowed vegetables.
You control the sodium level.
Use your favorite spices.
Always refrigerate and skim off any fat before using the broth.

Chicken Broth

Ingredients
200 grams skinless chicken meat chunks (breast preferred, no bones)
8 cups water
2 cups celery, cabbage, or fennel, sliced
1/4 onion, loosely chopped
2 tablespoons Bragg's liquid aminos
2 cloves garlic, crushed
1 tablespoon poultry seasoning
1/2 teaspoon garlic powder
1/2 teaspoon thyme
1/4 teaspoon mustard powder
Salt and pepper to taste

Makes 4-6 cups broth

.1 gram protein

<1 gram fat

<10 calories

PHASE 3
MODIFICATIONS:
Add additional
vegetables, meats
with bones, and spices
to create even more
flavorful broths.

Beef Broth

Ingredients
200 grams cubed beef (no bones)
8 cups water
3 tablespoons Bragg's liquid aminos
1 1/2 cups celery, sliced (substitute cabbage)
1/4 onion, loosely chopped
2 cloves garlic, crushed and minced
2 tablespoons salt or to taste
1 tablespoon peppercorns (substitute black pepper to taste)
1 teaspoon thyme
1/2 teaspoon marjoram

HCG DIET Tip

Make bundles of fresh and dried herbs and spices. Tie up herbs with string and add to soups or broth.

Vegetable Broth

Ingredients
Allowed vegetable (cabbage or celery)

8 cups water
2 tablespoons Bragg's liquid aminos
1 onion, loosely chopped
2 cloves garlic, crushed and minced
1 tablespoon peppercorns (substitute black pepper to taste)
1 teaspoon garlic powder
1/2 teaspoon mustard powder
Spices (your choice of spices such as thyme, rosemary, basil, etc.)
Salt and pepper to taste

Makes 4-6 cups broth
.1 gram protein
<1 gram fat
<10 calories

> Combine meats and/or vegetables with aminos, garlic, onion and spices. Simmer 1-2 hours, chill, skim off any fat, and use in soups or your favorite recipes. Makes approximately 6 cups of broth (use with allowed proteins/vegetables in soups and other recipes). Feel free to adjust the spices to your personal taste.

Variations: Save lean leftover meat from chicken or beef broth and add garlic, onion, other spices, and vinegar to create delicious chicken or beef salads. Serve over mixed greens.

Reuben Soup

Ingredients
100 grams lean corned beef
1/2 cup **Skillet Sauerkraut** (substitute fresh cabbage with additional
   vinegar and salt as desired)
1 1/2 cups water
1 1/4 cups beef broth
1 teaspoon apple cider vinegar
2 tablespoons minced red onions
1 clove garlic, crushed and minced
1/4 teaspoon caraway seeds

> Crush or roll caraway seeds and add to 1/4 beef broth and
> 1 teaspoon apple cider vinegar. Allow to marinate 30 minutes
> or more. Sauté onion and garlic with beef, then add caraway
> infusion. Rinse sauerkraut thoroughly. Add broth and water.
> Bring to a boil. Reduce heat and simmer for 20 minutes.

Makes 1 serving
(1 protein, 1 vegetable)
22 grams protein
8 grams fat
185 calories

PHASE 3
MODIFICATIONS: Top
with strips of Swiss
cheese.

Rosemary Chicken Soup

Ingredients
100 grams chicken breast, diced
1 1/4 cups chicken broth
1 1/4 cups water
1 1/2 cups celery, diced
1/4 teaspoon Bragg's liquid aminos
1 tablespoon onion, minced
1 clove garlic, crushed and minced
1/4 teaspoon mustard powder
1/8 teaspoon thyme
Salt and pepper to taste

> Sauté chicken, celery, onion and garlic in 1/4 cup chicken
> broth until lightly browned and liquid is absorbed. Add
> remaining broth, water and spices. Simmer for 20 minutes
> until celery is tender.

Makes 1 serving
(1 protein, 1 vegetable)
27 grams protein
2 grams fat
168 calories

Herbed Asparagus Soup

Ingredients

1 1/2 cups cooked asparagus
4 leaves fresh basil, rolled and minced
1/2 cup water
1/4 cup cooking water
1 tablespoon lemon juice
1 teaspoon Bragg's liquid aminos
1 teaspoon apple cider vinegar
1 clove garlic, crushed and minced
1 tablespoon onion, minced
1/8 teaspoon thyme
1/8 teaspoon marjoram
1/8 teaspoon mustard powder

Makes 1 serving
(1 vegetable)

5 grams protein

0 grams fat

65 calories

PHASE 3
MODIFICATIONS: Add
1/4 cup half and half, 1
ounce smooth melting
cheese.

> Cook asparagus in 1 1/2 cups water (or chicken broth if having
> chicken with that meal), and save out 1/4 cup cooking water.
> Puree cooked asparagus, basil, and spices with cooking water,
> aminos, lemon juice, and vinegar. Add 1/2 cup water and heat
> on low to medium heat for 3-5 minutes and serve.

Curried Beef Soup

Ingredients

100 grams beef, cubed
1 1/2 cups celery (substitute cabbage)
1 cup beef broth
1 cup water
1 teaspoon Bragg's liquid aminos
1 clove garlic, crushed and minced
1 tablespoon onion, minced
1 teaspoon curry powder
Pinch of pepper

Makes 1 serving
(1 protein, 1 vegetable)

22 grams protein

7 grams fat

175 calories

> Combine all ingredients and spices in a medium saucepan and bring
> to a boil. Reduce heat and simmer for 30 minutes until vegetables are
> tender. Add additional water or broth as needed.

Gingered Fennel Soup

Ingredients

2 cups fennel, chopped

1 1/2 cups water

1/4 cup vegetable broth (substitute chicken broth if you
   are cooking chicken for this meal)

2 tablespoons lemon juice

1 teaspoon Bragg's liquid aminos

1 clove garlic, crushed and minced

1 tablespoon fresh ginger, grated

1/8 teaspoon onion powder

1/8 teaspoon garlic powder

Pinch of lemon zest

Pinch of cinnamon

Pinch of pepper

Makes 1 serving
(1 vegetable)

3 grams protein

0 grams fat

70 calories

> Cook fennel in water approximately 7-10 minutes until tender.
> Drain fennel, saving 1/2 cooking water. Puree fennel and ginger
> with 1/4 cup vegetable broth. Add back to cooking water. Add
> spices and simmer for 7 minutes on low heat, stirring occasionally.

Savory Beef and Asparagus Soup

Ingredients

100 grams lean beef

1 1/2 cups asparagus spears, chopped

1 cup beef broth

1 cup water

2 tablespoons onion, chopped

1 clove garlic, crushed and minced

1/4 teaspoon thyme

1/8 teaspoon paprika

Salt and black pepper to taste

Makes 1 serving
(1 protein, 1 vegetable)

26 grams protein

7 grams fat

210 calories

> Sauté beef with onion in a little beef broth until lightly brown. Add
> broth, water, and spices and bring to a boil. Add asparagus, reduce
> heat and simmer for 20 minutes.

Hot and Sour Egg Drop Soup

Ingredients

1 1/2 cups water

1 whole egg, lightly beaten (eat 3 more egg whites
    to complete a protein serving)

2 slices lemon with rind

1-2 tablespoon Bragg's liquid aminos

1 tablespoon green onions, minced

1 teaspoon fresh ginger, grated

1 clove garlic, crushed and minced

1/8 teaspoon cayenne pepper

Pinch of Stevia to taste (optional)

Makes 1 serving
(1 protein)

7 grams protein

4 grams fat

82 calories

> Bring water with lemon, ginger, aminos and spices to a boil.
> Reduce heat and simmer for approximately 10 minutes until pulp
> from the lemons starts to come out. Remove the rind. Pour lightly
> beaten eggs in a thin stream while stirring in a circular motion for
> one minute. Top with green onions and serve.

Chilled Cucumber Soup

Ingredients

1 medium cucumber

2 tablespoons lemon juice

1 teaspoon Bragg's liquid aminos

2 tablespoons minced green onion

1-2 tablespoons fresh dill, chopped or 1 teaspoon dried

2 cloves garlic, crushed and minced

Makes 1 serving
(1 vegetable)

3 grams protein

0 grams fat

50 calories

> Puree ingredients in a blender. Chill and serve. Garnish
> with fresh dill and green onion.

Italian Wedding Soup

Ingredients
100 grams lean ground beef
1 1/2 cups fresh spinach
1 cup beef or vegetable broth
1 cup water
1 serving **Melba Toast Crumbs** (optional)
2 tablespoons onion, minced
1 clove garlic, crushed and minced
1/2 teaspoon basil, fresh or dried
1/4 teaspoon onion powder
Popcorn or Butter Flavor drops (optional)
Fresh parsley
Salt and pepper to taste

Combine ground beef, **Melba Toast Crumbs**, 1 tablespoon onion, onion powder, parsley, salt and pepper and form into meatballs. Bring broth and water to a boil. Add meatballs, additional onion, garlic, and spices to taste. Simmer for 25 minutes; add fresh spinach just before serving.

Makes 1 serving
(1 protein, 1 vegetable, 1 Melba toast)

23 grams protein	
8 grams fat	
188 calories	

PHASE 3 MODIFICATIONS: Substitute chicken broth (traditionally used in Italian Wedding Soup). Add additional vegetables such as carrots and celery. Top with parmesan cheese. Add 1/2 cup Shirataki pasta (orzo or chopped angel hair).

Gingered Shrimp Soup

Ingredients
100 grams shrimp, peeled
1 cup radishes, chopped (substitute spinach or cabbage)
2 cups water or vegetable broth
1 tablespoon Bragg's liquid aminos
1 tablespoon green onion, minced
2 slices lemon, with rind
1 clove garlic, crushed and minced
1 teaspoon fresh ginger, grated
Salt and pepper to taste

Bring broth to a boil. Add lemon and spices. Simmer for 10 minutes, then add shrimp and vegetables. Simmer for 10 more minutes, remove lemon rinds, and serve.

Makes 1 serving
(1 protein, 1 vegetable)

23 grams protein	
2 grams fat	
120 calories	

PHASE 3 MODIFICATIONS: Add fresh sliced mushrooms, additional vegetables (carrots, celery, zucchini, fresh broccoli).

Tomato Meatball Soup

Ingredients
100 grams lean ground beef
1 1/2 cups tomatoes, chopped
1 serving **Melba Toast Crumbs** (optional)
1/2 cup beef broth
1/2 cup water
1 tablespoon tomato paste
2 cloves garlic, crushed and minced
4 fresh basil leaves
1 tablespoon onion, minced
1/4 teaspoon paprika
1/4 teaspoon onion powder
1/4 teaspoon garlic powder
1/8 teaspoon thyme
1/8 teaspoon mustard powder
Pinch of nutmeg and clove
Pinch of black pepper
Cayenne pepper to taste
Stevia to taste
Salt and pepper to taste

Makes 1 serving
(1 protein, 1 vegetable,
1 Melba toast)

25 grams protein

9 grams fat

233 calories per serving

> Puree tomatoes, tomato paste, garlic, onion, and half of spices in a
> blender. Mix meat with **Melba Toast Crumbs**, the rest of the spices,
> and salt and pepper. Form into 3/4 inch-1 inch balls (makes about 7).
> Add broth and tomato mixture, bring to a boil. Reduce heat, simmer
> for 25 minutes, and serve.

Beef and Spinach Stew

Ingredients
100 grams lean steak or stew meat
1 1/2 cups spinach, loosely packed
2 cups beef broth
1 slice lemon with rind
1 clove garlic
2 tablespoons onion
1 teaspoon Italian herb mix
2 leaves fresh basil
Salt and pepper to taste

Makes 1 serving
(1 protein, 1 vegetable)
22 grams protein
8 grams fat
175 calories

> Slow cook beef in 1 3/4 cups beef broth, onion, garlic, and spices for
> 30 minutes uncovered (substitute 1 cup water to reduce sodium).
> Lightly steam spinach in 1/4 cup broth for one minute. Remove
> lemon slice, puree spinach and add to soup, then cook an additional
> 7-10 minutes, adding water as needed. Top with fresh basil and serve.

Variations: Substitute chicken and chicken broth.

Substitute: Chard for spinach.

HCG Diet Soup

Ingredients
2 cups water
1 1/2 cup cabbage, shredded (or other allowed vegetable)
2 tablespoons Bragg's liquid aminos
2 lemon slices with rind
1 clove garlic, crushed and minced
1 tablespoon onion, minced
Cayenne pepper to taste

Makes 1 serving
(1 vegetable)
1.5 grams protein
0 grams fat
50 calories

> Bring liquid ingredients to a boil. Add lemon, onion, garlic, cabbage,
> and spices. Simmer for 15 minutes and serve.

Salads

Fennel Salad with Mint

Wilted Beef and Spinach Salad

Sweet and Sour Cucumber Salad

Tomato Mint Salad

Teriyaki Slaw

Strawberry Spinach Salad

Sweet Curried Cucumber Salad

Chili Lemon Shrimp Salad

Apple Fennel Salad

Grapefruit and Chicken Salad

Sweet Shrimp and Asparagus Salad

Sweet Chili Radish Salad

Thai Beef Salad

Creamy Apple Salad

Taco Salad

Cajun Shrimp Salad

Smoky Fennel Salad

Fennel Salad with Mint

Ingredients
1 cup fennel, chopped
1/2 cup water
1 orange in segments
1 slice lemon with rind
2 tablespoons mint, crushed and minced
Pinch of cayenne
Stevia to taste

Makes 1 serving
(1 vegetable, 1 fruit)

2 grams protein

0 grams fat

105 calories

Chop fennel and prepare orange segments and mint. Set aside. To prepare the sauce, bring water to a boil with the lemon slice and three orange segments. Add cayenne and Stevia. Reduce heat and simmer until sauce is reduced. Remove the rind and blend flavors. Allow to cool and toss with fennel, mint, and orange slices. Chill and serve.

Wilted Beef and Spinach Salad

Ingredients
100 grams lean steak
1 1/2 cups spinach leaves, chopped

Dressing
Ingredients
1/2 cup beef broth
2 tablespoons apple cider vinegar
1 teaspoon lemon juice
1/8 teaspoon Bragg's liquid aminos
Few drops liquid smoke (to taste)
1 clove garlic, crushed and minced
Salt and pepper to taste

Makes 1 serving
(1 protein, 1 vegetable)

23 grams protein

8 grams fat

170 calories

PHASE 3
MODIFICATIONS: Add a little bacon/turkey bacon. Serve with fresh tomatoes.

Sauté beef in water and lemon juice with onions, garlic, aminos, salt and pepper until cooked. When liquid reduces and pan starts to brown, remove from heat. Deglaze the pan with beef broth and add vinegar and liquid smoke to taste. Add spinach and stir to wilt slightly in the pan. Top with beef and serve.

Sweet and Sour Cucumber Salad

Ingredients
1 medium cucumber, cubed
1 serving **Sweet and Sour Sauce**
Sliced oranges
1 tablespoon minced red or green onion

▶ Prepare **Sweet and Sour Sauce**, chill, and set aside. Prepare ingredients and assemble the salad. Chill and serve.

Makes 1 serving
(1 vegetable, 1 fruit)

4 grams protein

0 grams fat

110 calories

PHASE 3 MODIFICATIONS: Top with sesame seeds. Add additional vegetables such as red bell pepper and julienned carrots.

Tomato Mint Salad

Ingredients
1 1/2 cups tomatoes, chopped
1 tablespoon lemon juice
1 tablespoon mint, chopped
Pinch of black pepper
Stevia to taste

▶ Combine chopped tomatoes with mint, lemon juice, and Stevia. Toss lightly with a little Stevia and serve.

Makes 1 serving
(1 vegetable)

3 grams protein

0 grams fat

55 calories

Teriyaki Slaw

Ingredients
1 1/2 cups cabbage, shredded
Orange (remaining segments after preparing sauce)
1 serving **Teriyaki Sauce**
1 tablespoon green onion, minced

▶ Make **Teriyaki Sauce**, chill, and set aside. Prepare ingredients, utilizing the rest of the orange. Mix **Teriyaki Sauce** into cabbage and add onions and spices. Serve chilled.

Variations: Serve with chicken, beef, or shrimp.

Makes 1 serving
(1 fruit, 1 vegetable)

3 grams protein

0 grams fat

115 calories

PHASE 3 MODIFICATIONS: Add additional vegetables, top with sesame seeds.

Strawberry Spinach Salad

Ingredients
1 1/2 cups spinach leaves, washed and dried
5 strawberries
3 tablespoons water
2-3 tablespoons apple cider vinegar
1/4 teaspoon Bragg's liquid aminos
1 teaspoon finely minced onion
Pinch of cayenne pepper
Vanilla Stevia to taste (substitute a pinch of vanilla powder and
   regular Stevia)

Makes 1 serving
(1 fruit, 1 vegetable)

3 grams protein

0 grams fat

55 calories per serving

PHASE 3
MODIFICATIONS: Mix
dressing with a little
walnut, hazelnut, or other
oil. Add some almond
slices and a pinch of blue
cheese.

▶ Thinly slice 4 of the strawberries and set aside. Lightly mash or puree
   1 strawberry. Sauté onion, crushed strawberry, water, aminos,
   and Stevia until pan is lightly browned and water is absorbed. Turn
   off the heat and deglaze with apple cider vinegar. Stir to combine
   flavors and make a dressing. Add more Stevia to taste if desired.
   Toss dressing with spinach and the sliced strawberries and serve.

Sweet Curried Cucumber Salad

Ingredients
1 medium cucumber, sliced and quartered
1 apple, diced
1 tablespoon apple cider vinegar
1 tablespoon onion, minced
1/8 teaspoon curry powder or to taste
Stevia to taste

Makes 1 serving
(1 vegetable)

2.5 grams protein

0 grams fat

138 calories

▶ Combine vinegar and spices and blend, adding Stevia to taste.
   Toss dressing with cucumber, mix in minced onion, and serve.

Chili Lemon Shrimp Salad

Ingredients
100 grams shrimp, peeled
6 medium asparagus spears
2 tablespoons lemon juice
1 clove garlic, crushed and minced
1 tablespoon onion
1/2 teaspoon chili powder
Pinch of lemon zest
Stevia to taste
Salt and pepper to taste

Makes 1 serving
(1 fruit, 1 vegetable)

24 grams protein

1.5 grams fat

155 calories

> Lightly steam asparagus until crisp/tender. Cut into 1 inch pieces. Lightly steam shrimp until cooked. Allow to cool. Combine lemon juice, garlic, zest, and chili powder. Mix well and allow to marinate for 30 minutes in refrigerator and serve.

Apple Fennel Salad

Ingredients
1/2 apple, diced
1 cup fennel, diced (substitute raw celery)
1 serving **Melba Toast Croutons** (optional)
1 tablespoon lemon juice
1/2 teaspoon apple cider vinegar
1/8 teaspoon allspice
Pinch of black pepper (optional)
Stevia to taste

Makes 1 serving
(1 vegetable, 1 fruit,
1 Melba toast)

2 grams protein

0 grams fat

150 calories

> Lightly steam fennel until crisp/tender (about 5-7 minutes). Drain and toss with apple, lemon juice, and spices. Add **Melba Toast Croutons** and serve.

Grapefruit and Chicken Salad

Ingredients
100 grams chicken breast, cubed
1/2 grapefruit, segmented
1 1/2 cups Arugula or mixed greens
1/4 cup chicken broth
1 tablespoon lemon juice
1 serving **Sweet Onion Vinaigrette** or other compatible dressing

Makes 1 serving
(1 protein, 1 vegetable,
1 fruit)

26 grams protein

2 grams fat

200 calories

> Cook chicken breast with lemon juice until lightly brown. Deglaze the pan with chicken broth and stir until completely cooked. Toss with grapefruit, greens, and dressing, and serve.

Sweet Shrimp and Asparagus Salad

Ingredients
100 grams shrimp, peeled
1 1/2 cups cooked asparagus
1 orange
Juice from 2 orange segments
1 teaspoon lemon juice
1/4 teaspoon apple cider vinegar
3 leaves fresh basil, rolled and minced
1 tablespoon minced green onion
Pinch of black pepper

Makes 1 serving
(1 protein, 1 vegetable,
1 fruit)

26 grams protein

2 grams fat

230 calories

> Sauté shrimp in water until cooked. Steam asparagus. Combine orange juice, lemon juice, apple cider vinegar, basil, and pepper. Toss shrimp, asparagus and the rest of the orange with dressing and serve.

Variation: Enjoy with fresh minced tarragon. Substitute chicken breast or beef.

Sweet Chili Radish Salad

Ingredients
5 medium radishes (mild radishes taste best with this dish)
1 tablespoon lemon juice
1 teaspoon minced green onion
1/8 teaspoon (or a dash) chili powder
Stevia to taste

Makes 1 serving
(1 vegetable)

21 grams protein

8 grams fat

155 calories

> Slice or dice radishes. Add lemon juice, Stevia, and chili powder.
> Mix in green onion and lightly toss to coat.

Thai Beef Salad

Ingredients
100 grams lean steak, cut into strips
1 medium cucumber, thin sliced
2 red onion rings, quartered
2 tablespoons lemon juice
1 tablespoon Bragg's liquid aminos
1/2 teaspoon minced Thai Chili (substitute a pinch of red pepper
   flakes)
Pinch of fresh cilantro
Pinch of salt
Stevia to taste (optional)

Makes 1 serving
(1 protein, 1 vegetable)

23 grams protein

8 grams fat

189 calories

> Slice and prepare cucumber and onion. Sauté lean beef strips
> with a little salt to desired level of doneness. Remove from heat
> and assemble the salad. Combine ingredients and toss with
> aminos, lemon juice, cilantro and spices.

HCG DIET Tip

Spice up your soups, salads, and entrees with cayenne pepper. Cayenne pepper is believed to improve metabolism and be beneficial for weight loss as well as many other health benefits.

Creamy Apple Salad

Ingredients
100 grams nonfat cottage cheese
1 apple, cubed
1 cup celery, diced
1/8 teaspoon cinnamon
Vanilla Stevia to taste (or substitute plain Stevia and vanilla powder)

Makes 1 serving
(1 vegetable)

<1 gram protein

0 grams fat

15 calories

> Puree cottage cheese with Stevia and spices. Fold in apple and celery, and serve.

Taco Salad

Ingredients
100 grams lean ground beef
2 cups mixed green salad
1/4 cup water/beef broth
1 tablespoon onion, cut into strips
1 clove garlic, crushed and minced
1/8 teaspoon garlic powder
1/8 teaspoon cumin
Pinch of chili pepper/red pepper flakes
Salt and pepper to taste

Makes 1 serving
(1 protein, 1 fruit, 1 vegetable)

19 grams protein

.5 gram fat

195 calories

PHASE 3
MODIFICATIONS: Add chopped walnuts or almonds. Add other fruits such as grapes, or grated carrots.

Dressing

Ingredients
1 tablespoon apple cider vinegar
1 teaspoon Bragg's liquid aminos

> Cook ground beef with onion, garlic, and spices until beef is cooked and tender. Add beef to fresh salad greens. Add apple cider vinegar and aminos to pan drippings. Allow to cool and pour over salad.

Cajun Shrimp Salad

Ingredients
100 grams shrimp, peeled
2 cups mixed greens
1/4 cup water
2 tablespoons apple cider vinegar
1 tablespoon onion, minced
1/4 teaspoon Cajun seasonings

Makes 1 serving
(1 protein, 1 vegetable)

20 grams protein

1.5 grams fat

115 calories

> Sauté shrimp in water with Cajun seasonings and onion. Deglaze the pan with apple cider vinegar to create the dressing. Top mixed greens with shrimp and dressing, and serve.

Smokey Fennel Salad

Ingredients
1 cup fennel bulb, steamed and diced
1/2 teaspoon Bragg's liquid aminos
1 clove garlic, crushed and minced
Liquid smoke to taste (approximately 2-3 drops or 1/8 teaspoon)
1/2 teaspoon apple cider vinegar (optional)
1 tablespoon green onions, minced
1 tablespoon parsley, minced
Pinch of garlic powder
Pinch of onion powder
Pinch black pepper, freshly ground

Makes 1 serving
(1 vegetable)

1 gram protein

0 grams fat

32 calories

> Lightly steam fennel until crisp/tender. Add spices, lemon juice, and vinegar. Chill and serve.

Chicken Entrees

Sweet Chipotle Chicken Chili

Baked Chicken with Salsa Sauce

Savory Herb Lemon Chicken

Italian Chicken Nuggets

Spicy Chicken Loaf

Saffron Chicken

Chicken with Sage Citrus Sauce

Chicken Rosemary Casserole

Chicken Strips

Baked Chicken with Basil Asparagus Puree

Sweet and Sour Chicken Cabbage Rolls

Chicken with Lemony Cilantro Sauce

Chicken with Apple Fennel Sauce

Mediterranean Chicken Kabobs

Southwest Chicken Arugula

Chicken Molé

Baked Chicken Marinara

Chinese Chicken Stir Fry

Chicken with Spinach Pesto

Sweet Chipotle Chicken Chili

Ingredients

100 grams chicken breast
1/4 teaspoon chipotle chili powder (substitute regular chili powder
  if desired)
1 1/2 cups tomatoes, diced
1 cup water
1/2 cup chicken broth
1 tablespoon tomato paste
2 tablespoons onion, minced
1 tablespoon cilantro, chopped
1 clove garlic, crushed and minced
1/4 teaspoon garlic powder
1/4 teaspoon oregano
1/8 teaspoon cayenne pepper (or to taste)
1/8 teaspoon chili powder
Stevia to taste
Salt and pepper to taste

Makes 1 serving
(1 protein, 1 vegetable)

29 grams protein

3 grams fat

198 calories

PHASE 3
MODIFICATIONS:
Add bell peppers.

Sauté chicken with onion and garlic, until lightly brown. Add
tomatoes, broth, spices, and water. Simmer on low heat for
approximately 20 minutes or more, adding water as needed. Add
cilantro and Stevia to taste the last 5 minutes of cooking. Garnish
with cilantro.

Baked Chicken with Salsa Sauce

Ingredients
100 grams chicken breast
1 serving Melba toast
1 tablespoon lemon juice
1/8 teaspoon garlic powder
Pinch of cumin
Pinch of cayenne pepper
Salt and pepper to taste

Salsa Sauce

Ingredients
1 cup tomatoes, chopped
1 tablespoon cilantro, chopped
1 teaspoon lemon juice
1 tablespoon onion, minced
1 clove garlic, crushed and minced
1/4 teaspoon oregano
1/8 teaspoon cayenne pepper or to taste
Salt and pepper to taste

Makes 1 serving
(1 protein, 1 vegetable,
1 Melba toast)
29 grams protein
2 grams fat
194 calories

Crush Melba toast and mix in spices. Brush chicken with lemon juice and coat with Melba toast mixture. Bake at 350 degrees for 20 minutes until chicken is cooked. While the chicken is cooking, puree sauce ingredients in blender. Heat gently on low heat for approximately 3 minutes. Pour sauce over chicken and serve with additional tomato slices if desired.

Savory Herb Lemon Chicken

Ingredients
100 grams chicken breast
1 serving **Melba Toast Crumbs** (optional)
1/2 cup chicken broth
2 slices lemon with rind
1 teaspoon lemon juice
1/4 teaspoon Bragg's liquid aminos
1/8 teaspoon marjoram, fresh or dried
1/8 teaspoon thyme
1/8 teaspoon mustard powder or 1/4 teaspoon prepared mustard
5 Butter or Popcorn Flavor drops to taste (optional)
Salt and pepper to taste

Makes 1 serving
(1 protein, 1 Melba toast)

29 grams protein

2 grams fat

165 calories

PHASE 3
MODIFICATIONS: Add butter, capers, and white wine.

> Combine 1/2 cup broth with lemon slices with rind and spices. Simmer on low heat until liquid is reduced by half. Remove lemon rind and add Flavor drops. Dip chicken in lemon juice and coat with **Melba Toast Crumbs**. Bake at 350 degrees for 20 minutes or until chicken is cooked thoroughly. Pour sauce over the top and serve.

Italian Chicken Nuggets

Ingredients
100 grams chicken breast, cubed or diced
1 serving **Melba Toast Crumbs**
1/8 teaspoon Italian herb mix
Salt and pepper to taste

Makes 1 serving
(1 protein, 1 Melba toast)

26 grams protein

2 grams fat

155 calories

> Make **Melba Toast Crumbs** and add dry spices. Pat chicken dry, coat with **Melba Toast Crumbs** and arrange in single layer on baking sheet. Broil for approximately 5-7 minutes until chicken is cooked and nuggets are lightly browned.

Serving Suggestion: Serve with mustard, dressing, or **Strawberry Dipping Sauce**.

Variations: Try other spice combinations for more variety.

Spicy Chicken Loaf

Ingredients

100 grams chicken breast

1 serving **Melba Toast Crumbs** (optional)

1/2 teaspoon Bragg's liquid aminos

1 tablespoon onion, minced

1 clove garlic, crushed and minced

Pinch of red pepper flakes

Salt and pepper to taste

Sauce

Ingredients

3/4 cup tomatoes, chopped

1 tablespoon tomato paste

1 tablespoon cayenne pepper sauce (no sugar added sauce)

1 teaspoon apple cider vinegar

1/8 teaspoon garlic powder

1/8 teaspoon onion powder

Pinch of cayenne pepper (optional)

Stevia to taste

Salt and pepper to taste

Makes 1 serving
(1 protein, 1 vegetable,
1 Melba toast)

27 grams protein

2 grams fat

185 calories

PHASE 3
MODIFICATIONS: Add
red bell peppers and
green or black olives or
capers.

Pulse or grind raw chicken breast in food processor or bullet blender. Combine with onion, garlic and spices. Press chicken mixture into small loaf pan and bake at 350 degrees. Combine tomatoes, tomato paste with spices and puree. Pour over chicken mixture and bake at 350 degrees for 25-30 minutes.

Variations: Add a drop or two of Liquid Smoke for a BBQ flavor.

Saffron Chicken

Ingredients
100 grams chicken breast, cubed
1/2 cup chicken broth
2-3 tablespoons water or broth
1 tablespoon lemon juice
1 tablespoon onion, minced
1 clove garlic, crushed and minced
Pinch of saffron (a few threads is enough for one serving)
Pinch of red pepper flakes (optional)
Salt and pepper to taste

Makes 1 serving
(1 protein)

25 grams protein	
2 grams fat	
147 calories	

Lightly crush saffron and marinate in chicken broth with onion, garlic, lemon juice, and red pepper flakes for 10-20 minutes. Add saffron spiced broth mixture to chicken. Allow to simmer on low heat for 10 minutes until chicken is tender and liquid is absorbed. Allow pan to brown slightly then deglaze with additional 2-3 tablespoons of water or broth to create a sauce. Serve over a bed of steamed cabbage or spinach with a lemon wedge.

Variations: Add a pinch of cinnamon or ginger for added flavor.

Chicken with Sage Citrus Sauce

Ingredients
100 grams chicken
1 serving **Sage Citrus Sauce**
1 serving **Melba Toast Crumbs** (optional)
1 tablespoon lemon juice
2 tablespoons onion, minced
1 clove garlic, crushed and minced

Makes 1 serving
(1 protein, 1 fruit,
1 Melba toast)

25 grams protein	
2 grams fat	
175 calories	

Manually tenderize chicken and pound into flat patty. Dip in lemon juice and **Melba Toast Crumbs** and bake at 350 degrees for approximately 20 minutes or until chicken is cooked. Prepare **Sage Citrus Sauce** and pour warm sauce over chicken and serve.

Variations: Add apple cider vinegar to sauce and serve chicken over a green salad with oranges.

Chicken Rosemary Casserole

Ingredients
100 grams chicken breast, cubed
1 1/2 cups celery, diced
1/2 cup chicken broth
1 serving **Melba Toast Crumbs** (optional)
1 teaspoon Bragg's liquid aminos
1 tablespoon lemon juice
1 clove garlic, crushed and minced
1 tablespoon onion, minced
1/4 teaspoon rosemary
1/8 teaspoon mustard powder
1/8 teaspoon garlic powder
1/8 teaspoon onion powder
Pinch of cayenne pepper
Parsley
Salt and pepper to taste

Makes 1 serving
(1 protein, 1 vegetable,
1 Melba toast)

27 grams protein

2 grams fat

173 calories

Lightly sauté cubed chicken breast in 1/4 cup chicken broth until lightly brown. Set chicken aside and deglaze the pan with remaining chicken broth. Cook celery in 1/2 cup water until tender. Puree broth with cooked celery, rosemary and spices. Mix **Melba Toast Crumbs**, a pinch of additional crushed rosemary, salt and pepper. Combine chicken with celery mixture and top casserole with **Melba Toast Crumbs**. Bake at 375 degrees for 20-25 minutes. Top with parsley and serve with lemon wedges.

Chicken Strips

Ingredients
100 grams chicken
1 serving **Melba Toast Crumbs**, crushed
1 tablespoon lemon juice
1 teaspoon Bragg's liquid aminos
1/2 teaspoon apple cider vinegar
Pinch teaspoon oregano
Pinch chili
Pinch marjoram
Pinch paprika
Pinch onion powder
Pinch garlic powder
Pinch basil
Pinch sage
Salt and pepper to taste

Makes 1 serving
(1 protein, 1 Melba toast)

26 grams protein

2 grams fat

160 calories

PHASE 3
MODIFICATIONS: Bake
with **Marinara Sauce** and
provolone or serve with
sugar free dressing or
dip.

> Mix **Melba Toast Crumbs** with seasoning mix and set aside. Pound and flatten chicken breast and cut into strips. Marinate chicken in lemon juice and aminos for 20 minutes. Roll chicken in spiced Melba Toast mixture. Bake at 400 degrees for 10 minutes. Serve with **Strawberry Dipping Sauce**.

Tip: Flatten chicken strips in a bag and simply marinate in the bag.

Baked Chicken with Basil Asparagus Puree

Ingredients
100 grams chicken breast
1 1/2 cups asparagus, steamed
1 serving **Melba Toast Crumbs** (optional)
2 tablespoons chicken broth
2 tablespoons cooking water
1 tablespoon lemon juice
1 teaspoon Bragg's liquid aminos
6 leaves fresh basil
1 clove garlic
1/4 teaspoon garlic powder
Pinch of cayenne pepper

Makes 1 serving
(1 protein, 1 vegetable,
1 Melba toast)

35 grams Protein
3 grams fat
232 calories

> Steam asparagus until soft and set aside with 2 tablespoons of cooking water. Crush **Melba Toast Crumbs** and mix dry spices and a pinch of salt. Top chicken breast with Melba crumb mixture and bake at 350 degrees for 20 minutes. Blend asparagus with liquid ingredients, garlic, fresh basil, and cayenne pepper until smooth and creamy. Warm slightly in saucepan, pour over chicken and serve.

H C G
D I E T
Tip

To make a broth substitute that will work for most recipes, use 1 teaspoon Bragg's liquid aminos for each 1/4 cup of water called for in a recipe. Adjust your use of the Bragg's to your personal taste and personal sodium restrictions or requirements.

Sweet and Sour Chicken Cabbage Rolls

Ingredients
100 grams chicken breast
2-4 cabbage leaves
1 serving **Sweet and Sour Sauce**
1/2 cup water
1 clove garlic, crushed and minced
1 tablespoon onion, minced
Pinch of red pepper flakes
Stevia to taste

Makes 1 serving
(1 protein, 1 vegetable,
1 fruit)

27 grams protein

2 grams fat

210 calories

▸ Prepare one serving of **Sweet and Sour Sauce** and set aside. Lightly steam cabbage leaves and set aside. Mince or grind chicken breast in bullet blender with garlic, onion, and spices. Divide chicken mix into 2 servings. Double up, wrap and roll cabbage rolls with chicken mixture and place in baking dish. Add water to **Sweet and Sour Sauce** and pour over the cabbage rolls. Bake at 375 degrees for 30 minutes. Serve with warm **Sweet and Sour Sauce** poured over the top.

Chicken with Lemony Cilantro Sauce

Ingredients
100 grams chicken breast
1 serving **Lemony Cilantro Sauce**
1/4 cup chicken broth
1/4 cup water
3 slices lemon with rind
1 clove garlic, crushed and minced
6 cilantro leaves, fresh, minced
Pinch of Stevia (optional)
Salt and pepper to taste

Makes 1 serving
(1 protein)

26 grams protein

2 grams fat

145 calories

▸ Add chicken, garlic, and lemon slices to broth and water. Simmer for approximately 7 minutes until chicken is cooked and pulp is coming out of lemon slices. Remove rinds and add fresh cilantro leaves. Add more water or broth as needed and cook an additional 3 minutes until sauce is reduced and cilantro is infused into the sauce.

Chicken with Apple Fennel Sauce

Ingredients
100 grams chicken breast
1 cup fennel bulb, diced
1/2 apple, diced
3/4 cup chicken broth
2 tablespoons lemon juice
1/4 teaspoon garam masala sauce mix
Stevia to taste
Salt and pepper to taste

**Makes 1 serving
(1 protein, 1 vegetable,
1 fruit)**

27 grams protein

2 grams fat

212 calories

> Sauté chicken in 1/2 cup chicken broth until lightly browned and
> cooked. Cook fennel until very tender. Puree with diced raw apple,
> remaining 1/4 cup chicken broth, and spices. Heat gently on low heat
> for 1 minute. Serve over chicken and the rest of the apple on the side
> or thin slices on top.

Mediterranean Chicken Kabobs

Ingredients
100 grams chicken, cubed into 6 pieces
6 cherry tomatoes
Onion petals
1/4 cup chicken broth
Pinch of oregano
Pinch of mint
Pinch of basil
Pinch of lemon zest
Pinch of garlic powder
Salt and pepper to taste

**Makes 1 serving
(1 protein, 1 vegetable)**

28 grams protein

2 grams fat

170 calories

**PHASE 3
MODIFICATIONS:** Layer
with zucchini slices,
mushrooms, and brush
with olive oil.

> Marinate chicken in broth and spices for 1 hour or more. Soak skewers
> in water so they don't burn. Skewer chicken with onion and tomatoes,
> dividing ingredients in half to make 2 skewers, alternating ingredients.
> Broil or grill for 7-12 minutes, turning periodically until chicken is
> cooked and lightly browned. Serve with lemon wedges.

Southwest Chicken Arugula

Ingredients
100 grams chicken breast, cubed
1 1/2 cups arugula
3/4 cup chicken broth
1 tablespoon lemon juice
1/2 teaspoon apple cider vinegar
2 tablespoons onion, minced
1 clove garlic, crushed and minced
1/2 teaspoon cumin
1/8 teaspoon oregano
Fresh cilantro to taste
Salt and black pepper to taste

Makes 1 serving
(1 protein, 1 vegetable)

29 grams protein

2 grams fat

162 calories

PHASE 3
MODIFICATIONS: Add
tomatoes, zucchini and
other vegetables. Top
with sour cream and
cheddar cheese.

▶ Lightly sauté chicken in 2 tablespoons chicken broth until chicken and pan are lightly browned. Deglaze with remaining broth, lemon juice, and apple cider vinegar. Add onion, garlic, and spices and simmer until chicken is fully cooked and liquid is reduced by half. Lightly toss in arugula with chicken and sauce, and serve. Enjoy with additional arugula salad if desired.

Chicken Molé

Ingredients
100 grams chicken breast
1/2 cup tomatoes, chopped
1/2 cup chicken broth
2 tablespoons tomato paste
1 teaspoon apple cider vinegar
1 clove garlic, crushed and minced
1 tablespoon onion, minced
1/2 teaspoon chili powder
1/2 teaspoon defatted cocoa
Water as needed
Stevia to taste
Salt and pepper to taste

Makes 1 serving
(1 protein, 1 vegetable)

28 grams protein

2 grams fat

190 calories

▶ Sauté chicken with onion and chicken broth until lightly browned. Puree tomatoes with tomato paste, garlic, onion, vinegar and spices. Add to chicken and simmer on low heat for 25-30 minutes, stirring frequently and adding water as needed.

Baked Chicken Marinara

Ingredients
100 grams chicken breast
1 serving **Melba Toast Crumbs**
1 tablespoon lemon juice
1/4 teaspoon Italian herb mix
Salt and pepper to taste

Mix **Melba Toast Crumbs** with Italian herb mix, salt and pepper. Dip chicken breast in lemon juice and roll in herbed crumb mixture. Place in baking dish and bake at 375 degrees for 20 minutes until lightly browned and chicken is cooked. Pour **Marinara Sauce** over the chicken and serve.

Marinara Sauce

Ingredients
1 cup tomatoes (feel free to double, triple, or quadruple the recipe for multiple servings)
1 cup chicken broth
2 tablespoons tomato paste
1/4 teaspoon apple cider vinegar
2 cloves garlic, crushed and minced
2 tablespoons onion, minced
1 tablespoon basil, dried or fresh rolled (chop basil to taste)
1/4 teaspoon dried oregano
Pinch of marjoram
Pinch of Stevia
Salt and pepper to taste

Combine tomatoes, spices, and broth for sauce. Puree for smoother texture. Simmer on low heat for 30 minutes, stirring occasionally and adding water as needed to achieve desired consistency.

Makes 1 serving
(1 protein, 1 vegetable, 1 Melba toast)

30 grams protein	
2.5 grams fat	
251 calories	

PHASE 3
MODIFICATIONS: Top with cheese, mushrooms and chopped green or black olives.

Chinese Chicken Stir Fry

Ingredients

100 grams chicken breast, cubed
1 1/2 cups cabbage, cut in strips
1 cup chicken broth
2 tablespoons Bragg's liquid aminos
1 clove garlic, crushed and minced
2 tablespoons onion, chopped
1 teaspoon ginger, fresh, grated
Pinch of red pepper flakes
Water as needed

Makes 1 serving
(1 protein, 1 vegetable)
30 grams protein
2 grams fat
200 calories

PHASE 3
MODIFICATIONS:
Add mushrooms, bean sprouts, carrots, celery, and other Asian style vegetables.

▶ Fry chicken on high heat with 1/4 cup chicken broth until lightly brown. Add cabbage, the rest of the chicken broth, water and spices. Continue stirring, and turning ingredients until cabbage is tender, allowing water to evaporate and ingredients to brown slightly. Deglaze the pan by adding water as needed to create a rich sauce.

Variations: Substitute shrimp, beef, or celery; add oranges.

Chicken with Spinach Pesto

Ingredients

100 grams chicken breast
1 cup packed spinach
1 cup chicken broth
1 teaspoon lemon juice
1 teaspoon Bragg's liquid aminos
7 leaves fresh basil, rolled and minced
2 cloves garlic, crushed and minced
1/4 teaspoon garlic powder
Salt and pepper to taste

In a small saucepan, cook chicken with 1/2 cup chicken broth until liquid is absorbed and chicken is lightly brown. Set chicken aside and deglaze pan with 1/2 cup chicken broth. Add spinach and fresh basil and cook for 1 minute. Remove from heat. Puree spinach with garlic, lemon juice, aminos and spices. Add sauce to chicken, simmer 1-2 minutes and serve.

Makes 1 serving
(1 protein, 1 vegetable)
27 grams protein
2 grams fat
164 calories

PHASE 3
MODIFICATIONS: Add 2 teaspoons extra virgin olive oil, 1/4 cup walnuts or pine nuts, and 3 tablespoons parmesan cheese to the pesto mixture.

Beef Entrees

Beef with Herbed Fennel Puree

Roast Beef with Garlic Au Jus

Carne Asada Wraps

Beef and Cabbage Bake

Enchilada Pie

Picadillo Beef

Teriyaki Beef Kabobs

Smoky Beef Sausage

Curried Masala Beef Lettuce Wraps

Lemon Pepper Beef and Cabbage

Italian Beef Bake

Peppered Steak with Chard Puree

Beef with Sweet Mustard Sauce

Beef with Horseradish Sauce

Beefy Onion Boats

Chili Burgers

Beef with Herbed Fennel Puree

Ingredients
100 grams lean beef, sliced
1/2 cup beef broth or water
Salt and pepper to taste

Herbed Fennel Puree

Ingredients
1 cup fennel, steamed
1/2 cup beef broth
1 tablespoon lemon juice
1 teaspoon Bragg's liquid aminos
1 clove garlic, crushed and minced
1 teaspoon Italian herb mix
Salt and pepper to taste

Makes 1 serving	
(1 protein, 1 vegetable)	
22 grams protein	
8 grams fat	
187 calories	

Steam fennel until soft. Lightly salt and pepper beef. Sauté beef on medium heat with beef broth until lightly brown and liquid is absorbed. Deglaze the pan with beef broth and puree with steamed fennel, herbs, and liquid ingredients. Warm **Herbed Fennel Puree** and serve over beef.

HCG DIET Tip
Boil beef prior to cooking and drain off the fat. This is especially helpful if you are having trouble purchasing low-fat ground beef, etc.

Roast Beef with Garlic Au Jus

Ingredients
400 grams lean beef roast (round, sirloin, etc.)
  (14 ounce roast = 4 servings)
2 cups water
1/4 onion, chopped
4-6 cloves garlic, lightly crushed, cut in half
Salt and pepper to taste

Rub

Ingredients
1 teaspoon garlic powder
Add one pinch of each herb:
Thyme
Rosemary
Oregano
Basil
Marjoram
Salt and pepper to taste

Makes 4 servings
(1 protein each)

22 grams protein

9 grams fat

147 calories

PHASE 3
MODIFICATIONS: Add
vegetables to roast with
the juice. Use full fat
varieties of roast. Lightly
brown with olive oil on
all sides prior to slow
cooking.

Preheat oven to 250 degrees. Lightly brown the roast a few minutes on all sides in hot frying pan with a few tablespoons of broth. Cut 6-8 slits in the meat and add pieces of garlic. Coat roast with spice rub and sprinkle liberally with salt and pepper. Put 1 cup water in bottom of the pan and roast for approximately 1 1/2 - 2 hours or until an internal temperature of 160 degrees for medium. (Time will vary depending on your oven and the thickness of the roast.) Allow the roast to rest for 20 minutes, and then carve four equal servings. The pan will be dry.

To Make Au Jus:

Deglaze pan drippings with 1 cup water. Scrape the pan and dissolve the beef drippings. Chill the au jus, skim off fat. Serve with roast beef.

Carne Asada Wraps

Ingredients
100 grams lean flank steak
Large lettuce leaves for wrapping
3 tablespoons orange juice, fresh squeezed (eat remainder of orange
   to complete a fruit serving)
1 lemon, cut in wedges
1 tablespoon onion, crushed and minced
1 tablespoon fresh cilantro, minced
Pinch of cayenne pepper
Pinch garlic powder
Pinch of oregano
Salt and pepper to taste

Makes 1 serving
(1 protein, 1 vegetable,
1 fruit/optional)

22 grams protein

8 grams fat

160 calories

PHASE 3
MODIFICATIONS: Add
cubed avocado, cheese,
sour cream, and fresh
salsa.

▶ Marinate beef in orange juice and spices for a minimum of 30 minutes.
Sauté with a little water in a pan or BBQ until cooked and tender. Cut
into strips and enjoy with lettuce wraps. Serve with lemon wedges and
top with fresh cilantro.

Beef and Cabbage Bake

Ingredients
100 grams ground beef
1 1/2 cups cabbage, chopped
1/2 cup beef broth
1/2 cup water
2 tablespoons apple cider vinegar
1 tablespoon Bragg's liquid aminos
1 clove garlic, crushed and minced
1 tablespoon onion, minced
1/2 teaspoon caraway seeds
1/2 teaspoon garlic powder
1/8 teaspoon thyme
Pinch of paprika
Salt and pepper to taste

Makes 1 serving
(1 protein, 1 vegetable)

23 grams protein

8 grams fat

200 calories

▶ Brown ground beef with onion. Mix spices into broth and water.
Layer beef and cabbage in liquid. Sprinkle with paprika and pepper.
Bake at 375 degrees for 20 minutes.

Enchilada Pie

Ingredients
100 grams ground beef
1/4 cup beef broth
1 serving **Melba Toast Crumbs**
1 cup tomatoes, chopped
2 tablespoons tomato paste
2 tablespoons onions, minced
1 clove garlic, crushed and minced
1 tablespoon green onions
1/4 teaspoon chili powder
1/8 teaspoon oregano
1/8 teaspoon cumin
5 Popcorn or Butter Flavor drops (optional)
Salt and pepper to taste

Makes 1 serving
(1 protein, 1 vegetable,
1 Melba toast)

22 grams protein

8 grams fat

210 calories

PHASE 3
MODIFICATIONS: Top
with Monterey Jack or
cheddar cheese. Layer
with green ortega chilies.
Top with sour cream and
green onions, and serve.

▶ Puree broth, tomatoes, tomato paste, and spices. Brown ground beef with
onion and garlic. Pat off any extra oil. Mix **Melba Toast Crumbs** with salt
and Flavor drops. Combine beef and sauce, top with crumbs, and bake at
375 degrees until brown and bubbly. Top with green onions and serve.

Picadillo Beef

Ingredients
100 grams beef, minced or cubed
1 tablespoon tomato paste (eat fresh tomato to complete a
    vegetable serving)
1/2 cup beef broth
1/4 cup water
1/4 teaspoon apple cider vinegar
1 tablespoon onion, minced
1/4 teaspoon cumin
1/8 teaspoon garlic powder
1/8 teaspoon oregano
Cayenne pepper to taste
Salt and pepper to taste

Makes 1 serving
(1 protein, 1 vegetable)

22 grams protein

8 grams fat

157 calories

▶ Simmer beef, tomato paste, broth, water, and spices for approximately
15-20 minutes, adding water as needed until beef is tender.

Teriyaki Beef Kabobs

Ingredients
100 grams lean steak
1 serving **Teriyaki Sauce**
4 small onion petals
4-6 cherry tomatoes or other allowed vegetable
1 tablespoon green onions, minced

Makes 1 serving
(1 protein, 1 vegetable, 1 fruit)

23 grams protein

8 grams fat

180 calories

▶ Prepare **Teriyaki Sauce** and set aside. Soak skewers in water so they don't burn. Skewer cubes of beef with onion petals and tomatoes, dividing ingredients in half to make 2 skewers, alternating ingredients. Baste with **Teriyaki Sauce** and barbecue, bake, or broil to desired level of doneness, approximately 7-10 minutes, turning occasionally.

Smoky Beef Sausage

Ingredients
400 grams super lean ground beef
1 tablespoon apple cider vinegar
1 teaspoon Liquid Smoke
1 1/2 teaspoons garlic powder
1 teaspoon mustard powder
1/2 teaspoon salt
1/4 teaspoon cayenne pepper or to taste
1/4 teaspoon black pepper, freshly ground
Stevia to taste

Makes 4 servings
(1 protein)

20 grams protein

8 grams fat

145 calories

▶ Mix spices with ground beef. Separate into four 100 gram servings and refrigerate 4+ hours to blend flavors or cook up a fresh serving. Form patties for each 100 gram serving and fry with a little water in a small sauté pan until cooked.

HCG DIET *Tip* *Create your own lean ground chicken and beef by pulsing the meat several times in a food processor or bullet blender.*

Curried Masala Beef Lettuce Wraps

Ingredients
100 grams lean beef stew meat
4-6 lettuce leaves
1 cup beef broth
1 cup water
1 clove garlic, crushed and minced
1 tablespoon onion, minced
1/4 teaspoon curry
1/4 teaspoon garam masala spice mix

Makes 1 serving
(1 protein, 1 vegetable)
21 grams protein
7 grams fat
165 calories

> Simmer beef with liquids and spices on low/medium heat for approximately 20 minutes. Add water as necessary until beef is tender. Deglaze the pan with 1/4 cup water after pan browns to create the sauce. Serve beef with lettuce wraps or with other allowed vegetable.

Lemon Pepper Beef and Cabbage

Ingredients
100 grams lean ground beef or steak
2 cups cabbage, minced
1 cup beef broth
1/2 cup water (or more as needed)
2 lemon slices with rind
1 tablespoon onion, minced
1 bay leaf
1/8 teaspoon garlic powder
Black pepper, ground to taste

Makes 1 serving
(1 protein, 1 vegetable)
22 grams protein
8 grams fat
222 calories

> Brown the ground beef with the onion. Pat off any excess oil carefully. Sprinkle spices on the meat and add beef broth, bay leaf, and lemon slices. Bring to a boil and add cabbage and water. Sprinkle liberally with fresh ground pepper and simmer until water is absorbed and pan begins to brown. Add a little more water to deglaze the pan and continue cooking until cabbage is tender and most of the liquid is absorbed again. Remove lemon slices and bay leaf and serve hot. Garnish with a lemon wedge and additional black pepper.

Italian Beef Bake

Ingredients
100 grams lean ground beef
1 medium tomato, sliced
1/4 cup beef broth or water
1 tablespoon tomato paste
1 clove garlic, crushed and minced
3 basil leaves, rolled and minced
1 tablespoon onion, minced
1 teaspoon Italian herb seasoning mix
1/8 teaspoon garlic powder
Pinch of red pepper flakes (optional)

Makes 1 serving
(1 protein, 1 vegetable)

24 grams protein

8 grams fat

193 calories

PHASE 3
MODIFICATIONS: Add mushrooms, zucchini, bell pepper, and top with provolone/mozzarella cheese.

> Brown ground beef with onions and place in a medium baking dish. Top with sliced tomatoes and basil, garlic, and spices. Add broth and bake at 400 degrees for 25 minutes.

Peppered Steak with Chard Puree

Ingredients
100 grams lean steak
1 1/2 cups chard, cooked until tender
3 tablespoons beef broth or cooking water
1/2 teaspoon Bragg's liquid aminos
1 serving **Melba Toast Crumbs** (optional)
1/4 teaspoon oregano
1/8 teaspoon powdered mustard
Salt and pepper to taste

Makes 1 serving
(1 protein, 1 vegetable, 1 Melba toast)

23 grams protein

8 grams fat

217 calories

> Tenderize steak until pounded flat. Salt and pepper steak liberally and dip in **Melba Toast Crumbs**. Puree chard with garlic, onion, and spices and set aside. Bake steak at 375 degrees for 15 minutes or to desired level of doneness. Lightly warm chard puree on low heat and serve on top of steak or as a side dish.

Variations: Grill or fry steak. Serve chard puree over chicken breast or with seafood (use a different broth with the puree). Substitute spinach for chard.

Beef with Sweet Mustard Sauce

Ingredients
100 grams lean beef
1/2 cup water
1 teaspoon apple cider vinegar
1/2 teaspoon Bragg's liquid aminos
1 clove garlic, crushed and minced
1 tablespoon green onion, minced
3 slices fresh ginger
1 teaspoon powdered mustard
Stevia to taste

Makes 1 serving
(1 protein)

21 grams protein

7 grams fat

145 calories

> Sauté beef with ginger and onion until cooked. Add liquids and spices. Cook for approximately 10 minutes until liquid is reduced. Add additional cooking time and water as needed for more tender beef.

Variations: For a more savory dish, omit or use less Stevia and ginger and add savory herbs like rosemary or thyme.

Serving Suggestion: Serve in lettuce wraps or on a bed of steamed spinach or chard.

Beef with Horseradish Sauce

Ingredients
100 grams lean beef
5 radishes
2 tablespoons bottled horseradish (prepared without cream or sugar)
1 tablespoon Bragg's liquid aminos
1 tablespoon beef broth
1 tablespoon onion, minced
1 clove garlic, crushed and minced
Pinch of paprika
Pinch of mustard
Pinch of Stevia

Makes 1 serving
(1 protein, 1 vegetable)

22 grams protein

7 grams fat

160 calories

> Cook beef. Puree radishes, horseradish, liquids, and spices together. Warm sauce lightly in small saucepan and pour over beef or serve on the side.

Beefy Onion Boats

Ingredients
100 grams lean ground beef
1 cup beef broth
1/2 onion with center removed (makes a complete vegetable serving)
1 serving **Melba Toast Crumbs** (optional)
1/4 teaspoon thyme
1/8 teaspoon garlic powder
Pinch of rosemary
Pinch of cayenne pepper
Fresh parsley
Stevia to taste
Salt and pepper to taste

Makes 1 serving
(1 protein, 1 vegetable,
1 Melba toast)

23 grams protein

8 grams fat

192 calories

> Remove the center of the onion and use two medium sections to make the "Boats." Mince 1 tablespoon of the center of the leftover onion and mix into ground beef with spices and **Melba Toast Crumbs**. Pack this mixture into the center of the onion boats. Pour beef broth into the bottom of a small baking dish and layer with additional onion if desired, chopped or sliced into rings. Bake at 375 degrees for 30-40 minutes.

Chili Burgers

Ingredients
100 grams lean ground beef
1/4 cup beef broth
1/2 teaspoon lemon juice
1/4 teaspoon cayenne pepper sauce (no sugar added sauce)
1 tablespoon onion
1 clove garlic, crushed and minced
1/2 teaspoon chili
1/8 teaspoon garlic powder
1/8 teaspoon oregano

Makes 1 serving
(1 protein)

21 grams protein

7 grams fat

148 calories

PHASE 3
MODIFICATIONS: Top
with cheese or serve as
a salad.

Combine beef, liquid ingredients and spices and mix well. Form into patties and fry for 1-2 minutes on each side until burgers are cooked to desired level of doneness. Deglaze the pan with broth or water periodically to enhance the flavors or create sauce.

Variations: Form into meatballs and bake at 350 degrees for 20 minutes or add to soups.

Serving Suggestions: Serve with lettuce wraps or tomato slices.

Seafood Entrees

Fish Tacos

Mojito Shrimp

Dilly Fish Cakes

Baked Coconut Flavored Shrimp

Sweet Oolong Fish

Poached Fish with Wasabi Sauce

Fish with Dilled Asparagus

Crab Stuffed Cucumbers

Masala Fish

Asian Style Crab Cakes

Chipotle BBQ Shrimp

Shrimp Stuffed Tomatoes

Spicy Crab Bake

White Fish with Sweet Cucumber Relish

Crispy Cajun Shrimp

Fish with Dilled Tomato Sauce

Fish Tacos

Ingredients
100 grams white fish
4 large cabbage leaves
1 tablespoon lemon juice
1 serving **Melba Toast Crumbs** (optional)
1 tablespoon onion
Fresh cilantro
Pinch of cumin
Pinch of cayenne pepper
Pinch of oregano
Lemon wedges
Salt and pepper to taste

Makes 1 serving
(1 protein, 1 vegetable,
1 Melba toast)

22 grams protein

4 grams fat

178 calories

PHASE 3
MODIFICATIONS: Top
with salsa, avocado, sour
cream sauce, and chilies.

▶ Dip fish into lemon juice. Top with **Melba Toast Crumbs** mixed with spices. Bake at 425 degrees for 12-15 minutes or until fish is cooked. Serve in cabbage leaves and top with fresh cilantro, and onion. Serve with lemon wedges on the side.

Mojito Shrimp

Ingredients
100 grams shrimp, peeled
2 tablespoons lemon juice
1 teaspoon green onion, minced
Rum or Vanilla Flavor drops to taste
1 tablespoon mint leaves, fresh chopped
Pinch of lemon zest
Stevia to taste (optional)

Makes 1 serving
(1 protein)

20 grams protein

1.5 grams fat

105 calories

▶ Marinate shrimp in lemon juice and spices for 20 minutes. Sauté ingredients in a little water until shrimp are pink and cooked.

Variations: Serve Mojito Shrimp with **Tomato Mint Salad** or with lettuce leaves, taco style or as a salad.

Dilly Fish Cakes

Ingredients
100 grams white fish, minced raw
1 serving **Melba Toast Crumbs**
1 tablespoon lemon juice
1/2 teaspoon Bragg's liquid aminos
1-2 tablespoons fresh dill or 1 tablespoon dried dill
1 clove garlic, crushed and minced
1 tablespoon onion, minced
1/2 teaspoon Old Bay seasoning

Makes 1 serving
(1 protein, 1 melba Toast)

20.5 grams protein

4 grams fat

143 calories

> Finely mince or grind fish (or pulse in bullet blender). Mix in **Melba Toast Crumbs**, lemon juice, aminos, and spices. Form into patties and cook for 1-2 minutes on medium heat, turning periodically until fish is cooked. Deglaze the pan with a little water or lemon juice and serve. Garnish with fresh dill and lemon wedges.

Baked Coconut Flavored Shrimp

Ingredients
100 grams shrimp, peeled
1 serving **Melba Toast Crumbs**
1 teaspoon lemon juice
7 or more Coconut Flavor drops
5 Popcorn or Butter Flavor drops
Stevia to taste
Salt and pepper to taste

Makes 1 serving
(1 protein 1 Melba toast)

20.5 grams protein

1.5 grams fat

118 calories

> Remove tails from shrimp. Coat with lemon juice. Combine **Melba Toast Crumbs**, Flavor drops, and Stevia, and mix well. Dip shrimp in **Melba Toast Crumb** mixture and place in small baking dish. Preheat oven to 350 degrees and bake for 15 minutes or until shrimp is well cooked.

Sweet Oolong Fish

Ingredients
100 grams white fish
1/2 cup Oolong tea, strongly brewed
1 tablespoon Bragg's liquid aminos
1 tablespoon green onions, minced
1 teaspoon ginger, fresh grated
1 clove garlic, crushed and minced
Stevia to taste

Makes 1 serving
(1 protein)

21 grams protein

4 grams fat

125 calories

▷ Brew Oolong tea with ginger, garlic, onion, Stevia, and aminos. Marinate the fish in Oolong tea mixture in the refrigerator for 1+ hours. Sauté fish with marinade until fish is cooked and tender, and sauce is reduced by half. Top with green onions and serve with cabbage, spinach or other allowed vegetable.

Poached Fish with Wasabi Sauce

Ingredients
100 grams white fish
5 radishes
1/4 cup water
1 1/2 tablespoons Bragg's liquid aminos
1 teaspoon ginger, fresh
1 teaspoon white onions, minced
1 teaspoon green onions, minced
1/2 teaspoon garlic powder
1/4 powdered or prepared wasabi

Makes 1 serving
(1 protein, vegetable)

22 grams protein

4 grams fat

137 calories

▷ Poach fish in water or vegetable broth. Puree raw radishes with water, wasabi powder, aminos, onion, ginger, and spices. Lightly warm sauce and pour over fish. Top with green onions. Serve with lemon slices, additional fresh ginger, and aminos.

Serving Suggestion: Serve fish with a simple dipping sauce of aminos and a pinch of wasabi powder and ginger or substitute regular raw horseradish.

Fish with Dilled Asparagus

Ingredients
100 grams white fish
6-8 medium asparagus spears
1 serving **Melba Toast Crumbs**
1/2 cup water
1 tablespoon Bragg's liquid aminos
1 clove garlic, crushed and minced
2 tablespoons dill, fresh chopped
1 tablespoon lemon juice
1/8 teaspoon mustard powder
Lemon wedges
Salt and pepper to taste

Makes 1 serving
(1 protein, 1 vegetable,
1 Melba Toast)

26 grams protein

4 grams fat

195 calories

> Coat fish with **Melba Toast Crumbs** and bake at 425 degrees for 12-15 minutes or until fish is cooked and flaky. Sauté asparagus in water, aminos, lemon juice, garlic, onion, and dry spices until lightly tender. Toss asparagus with fresh dill, serve with fish, and garnish with lemon wedges.

Crab Stuffed Cucumbers

Ingredients
100 grams crab, steamed (substitute 75 grams pre-cooked crab)
1 medium cucumber, cut in half lengthwise
1 teaspoon Bragg's liquid aminos
1/2 teaspoon cayenne pepper sauce (no sugar added sauce)
1 tablespoon dill, fresh minced
1 tablespoon onion, minced
1/8 teaspoon garlic powder

Makes 1 serving
(1 protein, 1 vegetable)

23 grams protein

1.5 grams fat

150 calories

PHASE 3
MODIFICATIONS: Mix
in 1-2 tablespoons
mayonnaise.

> Hollow out the center of the cucumber and mix crab with onion, dill, garlic powder, cayenne pepper sauce, lemon juice, and aminos to make filling. Preheat oven and stuff cucumber with crab mixture. Broil 2-5 minutes (do not overcook) and serve with additional pepper sauce and aminos.

Variations: Add a little Stevia for a different flavor combination. Serve chilled as a salad. Top with **Melba Toast Crumbs** before broiling.

Masala Fish

Ingredients
100 grams white fish
1 cup tomatoes, chopped
2 tablespoons vegetable broth or water
1 tablespoon lemon juice
1 tablespoon onion, minced
1/8 teaspoon garam masala or to taste
1/8 teaspoon garlic powder
Pinch of red pepper flakes/cayenne pepper
Pinch of curry powder
Pinch of Stevia (optional)
Salt and pepper to taste

Makes 1 serving
(1 protein, 1 vegetable)
22 grams protein
4 grams fat
160 calories

▶ Marinate fish with curry, garlic powder, lemon juice, and cayenne pepper for 30 minutes or more . Sauté onions and garlic in 2 tablespoons of vegetable broth or water. Add fish, garam masala, and tomatoes and continue to sauté approximately 10-15 minutes, adding water as needed.

Asian Style Crab Cakes

Ingredients
100 grams crab meat (substitute 75 grams cooked crab meat)
1 serving **Melba Toast Crumbs**
1 teaspoon Bragg's liquid aminos
1 tablespoon green onion, minced
1 teaspoon ginger, fresh grated
Pinch of cayenne pepper
Pinch of Stevia or to taste

Makes 1 serving
(1 protein, 1 Melba toast)
21 grams protein
1.5 grams fat
122 calories

▶ Combine crab meat with spices and lemon juice. Mix in **Melba Toast Crumbs**. Lightly fry crab cakes until cooked and lightly browned. Deglaze with a little water periodically to create a sauce and serve with lemon wedges.

Serving suggestion: Serve over a green or spinach salad with orange slices.

Chipotle BBQ Shrimp

Ingredients
100 grams shrimp, peeled

Chipotle BBQ Sauce

Ingredients
2 tablespoons tomato paste
1/4 cup water
1 tablespoon lemon juice
1 tablespoon apple cider vinegar
1 tablespoon onion
1 clove garlic, crushed and minced
1/4 teaspoon chipotle pepper powder or to taste
1/8 teaspoon garlic powder
1/8 teaspoon onion powder
3-5 drops Liquid Smoke or to taste
Pinch of cumin
Stevia to taste
Salt and pepper to taste

Mix sauce ingredients and simmer 5 minutes until liquid is reduced by
half. Sauté shrimp in BBQ sauce 3-5 minutes until cooked, adding
water as needed.

Variations: Grill or wrap in foil, substitute regular chili powder.

Serving Suggestion: Serve with a side of fresh sliced tomatoes.

Makes 1 serving
(1 protein, 1 vegetable)
22 grams protein
2 grams fat
132 calories per serving

Shrimp Stuffed Tomatoes

Ingredients

100 grams shrimp, peeled
1 medium sized tomato
1 teaspoon apple cider vinegar
1 teaspoon Bragg's liquid aminos
1 clove garlic, crushed and minced
1 tablespoon cilantro leaves, fresh chopped
1 tablespoon green onion, minced
1/4 teaspoon Old Bay seasoning
Pinch of cayenne pepper (optional)
Salt and pepper to taste

Sauce

Ingredients

Inside of tomatoes
1/2 teaspoon Bragg's liquid aminos
1/2 clove garlic, crushed and minced
1 teaspoon cilantro leaves, fresh chopped
Pinch of Old Bay seasoning
Pinch cayenne pepper (optional)

Makes 1 serving
(1 protein, vegetable)

23 grams protein

2 grams fat

140 calories

Hollow out tomatoes and set insides aside to make sauce. Mince shrimp and add spices. Stuff tomatoes with shrimp mixture and bake at 400 degrees for 25-30 minutes. Puree sauce ingredients in a blender just before, warming for 2-5 minutes and serve.

Variations: Top with **Melba Toast Crumbs** before baking.

Spicy Crab Bake

Ingredients
100 grams crab
1 1/2 cups fennel, soft cooked
1 serving **Melba Toast Crumbs** (optional)
1 cup water
1 tablespoon lemon juice
1 teaspoon Bragg's liquid aminos
1/2 teaspoon apple cider vinegar
1 clove garlic, crushed and minced
1 tablespoon green onion or chives, minced
1/2 teaspoon Old Bay seasoning
1/8 teaspoon mustard powder
8-10 Butter or Popcorn Flavor drops (optional)
Pinch of cayenne pepper or to taste
Salt and pepper to taste

Makes 1 serving
(1 protein, 1 vegetable,
1 Melba toast)

23 grams protein

2 grams fat

165 calories

> Puree fennel with aminos, apple cider vinegar, and lemon juice (pulse until blended and smooth). Add spices and puree to combine. Add crab to fennel mixture and pour into brûlée dish or small baking dish. Mix **Melba Toast Crumb** mixture with Flavor drops, salt and pepper. Top casserole with spiced **Melba Toast Crumbs** and bake at 375 degrees for 25 minutes. Top with green onion and serve with lemon wedges.

Variations: Garnish topping with paprika, extra Old Bay seasoning and cayenne pepper to **Melba Toast Crumbs**.

White Fish with Sweet Cucumber Relish

Ingredients
100 grams white fish
1/4 cup water or vegetable broth
Pinch of salt and pepper

Sweet Cucumber Relish

Ingredients
1/2 medium cucumber, diced
1 tablespoon apple cider vinegar
1 tablespoon lemon juice
1 teaspoon Bragg's liquid aminos
1 clove garlic, crushed and minced
1/8 teaspoon onion powder
Pinch of cayenne
Stevia to taste

Makes 1 or more servings
(1 protein, 1 vegetable)

22 grams protein

4 grams fat

148 calories

> Combine cucumber with liquids and spices and marinate for 20-30 minutes. Sauté fish in water with salt and pepper until cooked and tender. Top with **Sweet Cucumber Relish** and serve.

Crispy Cajun Shrimp

Ingredients
100 grams shrimp, peeled
1 serving **Melba Toast Crumbs**
1 teaspoon lemon juice
1/2 teaspoon Bragg's liquid aminos
1/2 teaspoon Cajun spices
Lemon wedges

Makes 1 serving
(1 protein, 1 Melba toast)
21 grams protein
1.5 grams fat
120 calories

Hot Cajun Dressing/Dipping Sauce

Ingredients
3 tablespoons apple cider vinegar
1 tablespoon lemon juice
1/4 teaspoon Old Bay or Cajun seasoning mix
Pinch of garlic powder
Pinch of onion powder
Cayenne pepper to taste
Salt and pepper to taste

<5 calories

Dip shrimp in lemon juice and aminos. Add Cajun spices and coat shrimp liberally with **Melba Toast Crumbs**. Bake at 400 degrees for 7 minutes or until shrimp is cooked thoroughly. Serve with lemon wedges.

Variations: Omit the **Melba Toast Crumbs** and serve scampi style with a tablespoon of onion, 1 clove of garlic, and 2 tablespoons water or vegetable broth. Sprinkle with additional Cajun spices.

H C G
D I E T
Tip

Change up the recipes in this book by using different proteins to expand the variety and flavors.

Fish with Dilled Tomato Sauce

Ingredients
100 grams white fish
1/4 cup water or vegetable broth
1/4 teaspoon Old Bay seasoning (or other seafood seasoning mix)
Lemon wedges

Makes 1 serving
(1 protein, 1 vegetable)
23 grams protein
4 grams fat
160 calories per serving

Dilled Tomato Sauce

Ingredients
1 cup tomatoes, chopped
1 teaspoon lemon juice
1/4 teaspoon Bragg's liquid aminos
1 clove garlic, crushed and minced
2 tablespoons fresh dill
1 tablespoon onion, minced
1/2 teaspoon Old Bay seasoning
1/2 teaspoon apple cider vinegar
1/8 teaspoon garlic powder

Marinate fish in lemon juice, aminos and 1/4 teaspoon Old Bay seasoning for 30 minutes. Puree tomatoes with dill, garlic, onion, 1/4 teaspoon Old Bay seasoning, spices and liquid ingredients. Cook fish with marinade and a little extra water or broth until tender and cooked. Lightly warm Dilled Tomato Sauce and pour over fish. Serve with lemon wedges and garnish with parsley and additional tomato slices if desired.

Variations: Serve sauce as a dipping sauce for shrimp or chicken.

Egg and Cheese Entrees

Spiced Cottage Cheese with Tomatoes

Breakfast Hash

Tomato Basil Bake

Cabbage Cheese Casserole

Italian Spinach Cheese Cups

Egg Salad

Caramelized Onion Tart

Florentine Scramble

Sage and Onion Cottage Pie

Curried Eggs with Tomatoes

Asparagus Casserole

Italian Spinach Frittata

Poached Eggs with Spicy Tomato Sauce

Spiced Cottage Cheese with Tomatoes

Ingredients
100 grams nonfat cottage cheese
2 medium tomatoes, sliced
1 tablespoon onion, minced
1/8 teaspoon cayenne pepper (or to taste)
1/8 teaspoon garlic powder
Fresh ground black pepper
Pinch of salt

Makes 1 serving
(1 protein, 1 vegetable)
20 grams protein
.5 grams fat
138 calories

▶ Mix spices into cottage cheese. Top with tomatoes and sprinkle with fresh ground pepper.

Variation: Serve with Melba toast. Top with a splash of cayenne pepper sauce.

Breakfast Hash

Ingredients
1 whole egg
3 egg whites
1 cup cabbage, chopped
1 cup water or broth
1/2 teaspoon Bragg's liquid aminos
1/2 teaspoon cayenne pepper sauce (no sugar added sauce)
1 tablespoon onion, minced
1/4 teaspoon garlic powder
1/4 teaspoon (Italian herbs, thyme, or other spice mix)
Salt and pepper to taste

Makes 1 serving
(1 protein, 1 vegetable)
19 grams protein
4 grams fat
168 calories

PHASE 3
MODIFICATIONS:
Add breakfast meat
(like bacon or sausage)
or cheese.

▶ Sauté cabbage with liquids and spices until cabbage is tender and liquid is absorbed. Add lightly beaten eggs and stir until ingredients are combined and eggs are cooked.

Note: Some varieties of cabbage cook more slowly. Feel free to add more water as needed.

Tomato Basil Bake

Ingredients
100 grams nonfat cottage cheese
1 cup tomatoes, chopped
1 serving **Melba Toast Crumbs**
5 leaves fresh basil, rolled and minced
1 clove garlic, crushed and minced
1 tablespoon onion, minced
1/8 teaspoon garlic powder
1/8 teaspoon thyme
Salt and pepper to taste

Makes 1 serving
(1 protein, 1 vegetable,
1 Melba toast)

18 grams protein

.5 gram fat

142 calories

> Puree cottage cheese, tomatoes, and spices in a blender or food processor until smooth. Stir in onion, 1/2 **Melba Toast Crumbs** and pour into small baking dish. Top with remaining crumbs and bake at 400 degrees for 25 minutes until bubbly.

Cabbage Cheese Casserole

Ingredients
100 grams nonfat cottage cheese
1 cup cabbage, chopped
1 serving **Melba Toast Crumbs**
1/2 teaspoon Bragg's liquid aminos
1 clove garlic, crushed and minced
1 tablespoon onion, minced
1/8 teaspoon onion powder
1/8 teaspoon garlic powder
1/8 teaspoon thyme

Makes 1 serving
(1 protein, 1 vegetable,
1 Melba toast)

20 grams protein

1 gram fat

142 calories

> Puree cottage cheese with raw cabbage, aminos, onion, garlic and spices, and pour into baking dish. Top with **Melba Toast Crumbs** and bake at 400 degrees for 25 minutes.

Italian Spinach Cheese Cups

Ingredients
100 grams nonfat cottage cheese
1 cup spinach, chopped
1 serving **Melba Toast Crumbs**
1 tablespoon milk
1 teaspoon Bragg's liquid aminos
1/2 teaspoon Italian herb spice mix
1/8 teaspoon garlic powder
1/8 teaspoon onion powder
Pinch of cayenne pepper or to taste
Salt and pepper to taste

Makes 1 serving (1 protein, 1 vegetable, 1 Melba Toast)
20 grams protein
1 gram fat
127 calories

> Puree spinach and cottage cheese with spices and 1 tablespoon milk. Stir in1/2 of **Melba Toast Crumbs** and mix well. Pour into small baking dish, sprinkle with the rest of **Melba Toast Crumbs** and bake at 400 degrees for 25 minutes.

Egg Salad

Ingredients
4 eggs
1 teaspoon Bragg's liquid aminos
1 teaspoon apple cider vinegar
1 tablespoon onion, minced (green onion is best)
Pinch of paprika
Cayenne pepper to taste (optional)
Salt and pepper to taste

Makes 1 serving (1 protein)
18 grams protein
4 grams fat
132 calories

> Boil eggs for 10-15 minutes (10 minutes for medium eggs, up to 15 minutes for large eggs). Drain eggs and remove shell. Discard 3 of the yolks (one yolk is allowed per protein serving). Chop eggs into medium pieces, add spices and liquids, and mix well. Serve over a bed of salad greens.

Caramelized Onion Tart

Ingredients
1 whole egg
3 egg whites
1/2 cup onions (makes a complete vegetable serving)
4 tablespoons water
1 tablespoon milk (optional)
1 tablespoon lemon juice
1/2 teaspoon Bragg's liquid aminos
Pinch of onion powder
Pinch of marjoram
Pinch of cayenne pepper
Vanilla or English Toffee Stevia to taste
Salt and pepper to taste

Makes 1 serving
(1 protein, 1 vegetable)

18 grams protein

4 grams fat

165 calories

PHASE 3
MODIFICATIONS: Top
with Gruyere or Swiss
cheese strips.

Lightly beat eggs with milk and spices to taste. Lightly sauté onions with Stevia, 2 tablespoons water, lemon juice, and aminos until tender. Allow to brown and then remove from heat and deglaze with remaining 2 tablespoons of water. Layer onions on the bottom of small baking dish and pour in egg mixture. Bake at 375 degrees for 25 minutes. Allow to set for 2-5 minutes and enjoy.

Florentine Scramble

Ingredients
1 whole egg
3 egg whites
1 cup spinach, sliced into strips
2 tablespoons water
1 tablespoon milk
1/2 teaspoon Bragg's liquid aminos
1 clove garlic, crushed and minced
1 tablespoon onion, minced
5 -7 Popcorn or Butter Flavor drops
Pinch nutmeg
Salt and pepper to taste

Makes 1 serving
(1 protein, 1 vegetable)

20 grams protein

4 grams fat

149 calories

PHASE 3
MODIFICATIONS: Add
grated gruyere cheese or
other cheese.

Lightly beat eggs with milk, garlic, and dried spices. Sauté spinach, onion, and garlic with water and aminos. Add eggs, scramble, and serve.

Sage and Onion Cottage Pie

Ingredients
100 grams nonfat cottage cheese
2 tablespoons onion, chopped
3 onion rings (makes a complete vegetable serving)
1 serving **Melba Toast Crumbs**
1 clove garlic, crushed and minced
1/8 teaspoon garlic powder
1/8 teaspoon onion powder
1/8 teaspoon powered sage or 3 leaves sage, rolled and finely minced
  (optional)
Pinch of paprika
Pinch of salt
Pinch of Stevia
Cayenne pepper to taste

Makes 1 serving
(1 protein, 1 vegetable,
1 Melba toast)

18 grams protein

1 gram fat

110 calories

▶ Layer 3 onion rings in a brûlée or small baking dish. Puree cottage cheese, chopped onion, and spices and mix well. Stir in 1/2 of **Melba Toast Crumbs**. Top onion rings with spiced cottage cheese mixture and sprinkle with additional sage, and rest of **Melba Toast Crumbs**. Bake at 400 degrees for 20 minutes until lightly browned on top.

Curried Eggs with Tomatoes

Ingredients
1 whole egg
3 egg whites, beaten
1 cup tomato, chopped or 6 cherry tomatoes, halved
1 tablespoon green onion, minced
1/2 teaspoon curry powder
Stevia to taste

Makes 1 serving
(1 protein, 1 vegetable)

19 grams protein

4 grams fat

165 calories

▶ Add curry powder and Stevia to beaten eggs. Scramble eggs with tomatoes and onion until cooked. Top with minced green onion and serve.

Asparagus Casserole

Ingredients
1 whole egg
3 egg whites
1 1/2 cups asparagus, chopped
3 tablespoons water
1 tablespoon milk
1 teaspoon Bragg's liquid aminos
1 tablespoon onion, minced
1 clove garlic, crushed and minced
1/4 teaspoon thyme
Salt and pepper to taste

Makes 1 serving
(1 protein, 1 vegetable)

21 grams protein

4 grams fat

190 calories

PHASE 3
MODIFICATIONS: Top
with grated cheddar
cheese. Mix in 2
tablespoons parmesan
cheese.

> Steam and puree asparagus with 3 tablespoons water. Lightly
> beat egg whites with milk. Fold in asparagus puree and add
> spices. Bake at 375 degrees for 25 minutes.

Italian Spinach Frittata

Ingredients
1 whole egg
3 egg whites
1 cup spinach, chopped
1 tablespoon milk (optional)
1 clove garlic, crushed and minced
1 tablespoon onion, minced
1/2 teaspoon Italian herbs
1/4 teaspoon thyme
1/8 teaspoon garlic powder
1/8 teaspoon onion powder
Cayenne pepper to taste (optional)
Salt and pepper to taste

Makes 1 serving
(1 protein, 1 vegetable)

19 grams protein

4 grams fat

150 calories

> Lightly beat eggs with milk, onion, garlic, and spices. Pour mixture
> into small baking dish. Add spinach and bake at 375 degrees for
> 20 minutes.

Poached Eggs with Spicy Tomato Sauce

Ingredients
1 whole egg
3 egg whites
3/4 cup water
1 teaspoon apple cider vinegar for poaching

Spicy Tomato Sauce

Ingredients
1 large tomato, chopped
1 tablespoon tomato paste
1 tablespoon apple cider vinegar
1 clove garlic, crushed and minced
1 tablespoon cilantro, minced
1 tablespoon onion, minced
Pinch of onion powder
Pinch of garlic powder
Pinch of cayenne pepper or to taste
Salt and pepper to taste

Makes 1 serving
(1 protein, 1 vegetable)

20 grams protein

4 grams fat

190 calories

PHASE 3
MODIFICATIONS: Serve
with sour cream and/or
cheese.

> To make spicy tomato sauce, puree tomato, tomato paste, garlic, onion, cilantro and spices in food processor or bullet blender. Poach eggs in water and vinegar to desired level of doneness (3 minutes for medium, 4-5 for well done). Remove eggs from water, warm sauce, pour over poached eggs and serve.

HCG
DIET
Tip

Save 1 egg white to make some meringue cookies to enjoy as a snack.

Vegetables

Garlic Fennel Mash

Sweet Apple Cabbage

Gingered Chard Sauté

Roasted Garlic Asparagus

Lemon Pepper Spinach

Savory Celery

Braised Tarragon Fennel

Veggies with Sweet Mustard Dip

Sautéed Mustard Radishes

Skillet Sauerkraut

Orange and Sage Asparagus

Asian Spinach Sauté

Orange Rosemary Fennel

Sweet and Sour Cabbage

Lemon Ginger Asparagus

Broiled Basil Tomatoes

Sweet and Spicy Apple Chard

Garlic Fennel Mash

Ingredients
1 1/2 cups fennel, soft cooked
1 tablespoon milk
1 teaspoon Bragg's liquid aminos
2 cloves garlic, crushed and minced
1/2 teaspoon garlic powder
5 drops Popcorn or Butter Flavor drops (optional)
Salt and pepper to taste

Makes 1 serving
(1 vegetable)

2 grams protein

0 grams fat

50 calories

▶ Puree fennel, add garlic, aminos, lemon juice, and Flavor drops to spices.
Heat in small sauce pan. Top with minced green onion (optional).

Variations: Add Italian herb mix or fresh dill and serve with fish or chicken.

Sweet Apple Cabbage

Ingredients
1 apple, cubed
1 1/2 cups cabbage
1 cup water
3 tablespoons apple cider vinegar
1 tablespoon lemon juice
Pinch of marjoram
Stevia to taste
Salt and pepper to taste

Makes 1 serving
(1 vegetable, 1 fruit)

2 grams protein

0 grams fat

140 calories

▶ Simmer cabbage in water, vinegar, and spices for 5-7 minutes.
Add cubed apple and cook for an additional 7 minutes, stirring
frequently and adding water as needed. Add Stevia to taste and
extra lemon juice if desired.

Gingered Chard Sauté

Ingredients
1 1/2 cups chard
1/2 cup water
2 tablespoons lemon juice
1 tablespoon Bragg's liquid aminos
2 cloves garlic, crushed and minced
1 tablespoon green onion
1 teaspoon ginger, fresh grated
Pinch of red pepper flakes (optional)
Pinch of Stevia

Makes 1 serving
(1 vegetable)

3 grams protein

0 grams fat

54 calories

> Sauté chard with liquids and spices. Cook until tender.
> Add water as needed.

Roasted Garlic Asparagus

Ingredients
6 medium spears asparagus
1/2 cup water or broth (use broth for a protein for that meal)
1 teaspoon Bragg's liquid aminos
2 cloves garlic, crushed and minced
1/4 teaspoon thyme
1/8 teaspoon mustard powder
Salt and pepper to taste

Makes 1 serving
(1 vegetable)

1 gram protein

0 grams fat

60 calories

> Sauté garlic with 1/4 cup water or broth, aminos, and spices until
> liquid is absorbed and pan begins to brown. Deglaze the pan with
> remaining broth and add asparagus. Cover and simmer until
> asparagus is tender, adding water as needed to create more sauce.
> Spoon garlic sauce over asparagus and serve.

Lemon Pepper Spinach

Ingredients
1 1/2 cups spinach leaves
1/4 cup water
1/4 cup broth (chicken, beef, or vegetable depending on what protein
   you are using)
2 lemon slices with rind
1 clove garlic, crushed and minced
1 tablespoon onion, minced
Salt and pepper to taste

Makes 1 serving
(1 vegetable)

2 grams protein

0 grams fat

32 calories per serving

PHASE 3
MODIFICATIONS: Add 1
tablespoon olive oil.

▶ Sauté lemon slices, garlic, and onion in broth and water for
approximately five minutes. Remove the lemon rinds. Add spinach,
spice and water as needed. Lightly cook, and serve.

Savory Celery

Ingredients
1 1/2 cups celery
1 1/2 cups water
1 tablespoon Bragg's liquid aminos
1/2 teaspoon apple cider vinegar
1 slice of lemon with rind
2 cloves garlic, crushed and minced
1/4 teaspoon thyme
Salt and pepper to taste

Makes 1 serving
(1 vegetable)

1 gram protein

0 grams fat

27 calories

▶ Cover and cook celery in 1 1/4 cups water with slice of lemon, garlic,
thyme and aminos until tender, water is absorbed and pan is starting
to brown. Add 1/4 cup more water to deglaze the pan. Add apple cider
vinegar, sprinkle of paprika, and serve.

Braised Tarragon Fennel

Ingredients

1/2 medium bulb fennel, cut into wedges

1/2 cup vegetable broth (substitute chicken or beef broth if you are serving with those proteins)

1/2 teaspoon Bragg's liquid aminos

1 tablespoon tarragon, fresh or dried minced (fresh is recommended)

1 tablespoon lemon juice

1/8 teaspoon garlic powder

Salt and pepper to taste

Makes 1 serving
(1 vegetable)

.5 grams protein

0 grams fat

25 calories

▶ Halve the fennel bulb and cut into thin wedges (6-8). Layer in a small, low baking dish and sprinkle with garlic powder, lemon juice, aminos, salt, and pepper. Pour broth into baking dish (about halfway to fennel wedges). Sprinkle with fresh tarragon. Bake at 375 degrees for 25 minutes or until tender.

Veggies with Sweet Mustard Dip

Ingredients

1 1/2 cups allowed vegetables, raw chopped (radishes, cucumber, or celery)

1/4 cup water

1 teaspoon Bragg's liquid aminos

1/2 teaspoon apple cider vinegar

3 slices fresh ginger

1 tablespoon red onion, minced

1/2 teaspoon mustard powder

1/4 teaspoon garlic powder

Stevia to taste

Makes 1 serving
(1 vegetable)

1 gram protein

0 grams fat

25 calories

▶ Prepare vegetables and set aside. Combine spices and liquids and heat gently for 1-2 minutes until sauce is reduced. Set aside and allow to cool. Use as a dipping sauce for vegetables.

Variations: Add additional vinegar to make salad dressing or mix into spinach or other greens.

Sautéed Mustard Radishes

Ingredients
5 radishes, sliced
1/4 cup water
1/2 teaspoon apple cider vinegar
1/2 teaspoon Bragg's liquid aminos
1 tablespoon prepared mustard
1 tablespoon red onion, minced
Fresh ginger – 3 slices
1/4 teaspoon garlic powder
Stevia to taste

Makes 1 serving
(1 vegetable)

1 gram protein	
0 grams fat	
18 calories	

▶ Sauté radishes with mustard, apple cider vinegar, onion, garlic, aminos, and ginger until tender and sauce is reduced by half.

Skillet Sauerkraut

Ingredients
2 cups cabbage, shredded
2 1/2 cups water
3 slices lemon
1/2 teaspoon apple cider vinegar
1 teaspoon salt

Makes 1 serving
(1 vegetable)

1.5 grams protein	
0 grams fat	
50 calories	

▶ Boil lemon, salt, and vinegar for 5 minutes. Add cabbage and cook for approximately 15 minutes until liquid is absorbed. Remove lemon slices and add additional salt and vinegar for an even tangier flavor if desired.

Orange and Sage Asparagus

Ingredients
6-8 medium spears asparagus
1 serving **Sage Citrus Sauce**
3 segments orange
1 tablespoon red onion, minced
1 teaspoon sage, fresh minced (optional)
Salt and pepper to taste

Makes 1 serving
(1 vegetable, 1 fruit)

5 grams protein	
0 grams fat	
130 calories	

▶ Prepare **Sage Citrus Sauce** and set aside. Lightly steam asparagus until crisp/tender. Toss asparagus with sauce, onions, orange segments, and fresh sage. Serve hot or chilled.

Asian Spinach Sauté

Ingredients
1 1/2 cups spinach, chopped
1/4 cup water or vegetable broth
1 tablespoon Bragg's liquid aminos
1 clove garlic, crushed and minced
1 tablespoon onion, minced
1 teaspoon apple cider vinegar
1/4 teaspoon ginger, fresh minced
Stevia to taste (optional)
Salt and pepper to taste

Makes 1 serving
(1 vegetable)

3 grams protein

0 grams fat

30 calories

PHASE 3
MODIFICATIONS: Drizzle
with a little sesame oil
and top with sesame
seeds.

> Sauté onion, garlic, and ginger in aminos and a little water until pan begins to brown. Deglaze the pan with water or broth. Remove from heat and add spinach. Sauté 1-3 minutes and serve.

Orange Rosemary Fennel

Ingredients
1/2 fennel bulb, cut into thin wedges
1/2 orange, cubed (eat the rest of the orange to make
   a complete fruit serving)
1 serving **Melba Toast Crumbs** (optional)
3/4 cup water or vegetable broth
1 tablespoon lemon juice
1 tablespoon red onion, minced
1/2 teaspoon rosemary
Pinch of lemon zest
Salt and pepper to taste

Makes 1 serving
(1 vegetable, 1 fruit,
1 Melba toast)

2 grams protein

0 grams fat

95 calories

> Layer fennel wedges in a single layer in small baking pan, top with oranges, rosemary, onion, and **Melba Toast Crumbs**. Bake at 400 degrees for 25 minutes until tender.

Sweet and Sour Cabbage

Ingredients

1 1/2 cups cabbage, loosely chopped

1 serving **Sweet and Sour Sauce** (eat the rest of the orange
  to complete a fruit serving)

1 1/2 cups water

1 clove garlic, crushed and minced

1 tablespoon onion, minced

Makes 1 serving
(1 vegetable, 1 fruit)

3 grams protein

0 grams fat

77 calories

▷ Prepare cabbage, add water, garlic, onions, and **Sweet and Sour Sauce**. Simmer covered on low heat until liquid is gone and cabbage is tender. Deglaze with a little more water, stir, and serve.

Lemon Ginger Asparagus

Ingredients

6-8 medium spears asparagus

1 serving **Sweet Lemon Ginger Sauce**

Pinch of lemon zest

Stevia to taste

Salt and pepper to taste

Makes 1 serving
(1 vegetable)

5 grams protein

0 grams fat

62 calories

PHASE 3
MODIFICATIONS: Add
1/2 tablespoon butter to
the sauce and top with
a tablespoon of sliced
almonds.

▷ Prepare **Sweet Lemon Ginger Sauce** and set aside. Steam asparagus until crisp/tender. Toss with sauce or pour over the top and serve. Garnish with lemon slices.

HCG
DIET
Tip

Plan your meals in advance and take a weekly trip to the grocery store or farmers market for fresh meats and produce.

Broiled Basil Tomatoes

Ingredients
1 medium tomato, cut in half
1 serving **Melba Toast Crumbs**
1/4 cup water
1 clove garlic, crushed and minced
4 leaves fresh basil, rolled and minced
1 tablespoon onion, minced
1/8 teaspoon garlic powder
Fresh parsley
Salt and pepper to taste

Makes 1 serving
(1 vegetable, 1 Melba toast)

3 grams protein

0 grams fat

63 calories

PHASE 3 MODIFICATIONS: Top with a little grated parmesan, provolone, or mozzarella cheese.

Place tomato halves in small baking dish with water. Make **Melba Toast Crumbs** and add garlic powder, salt, spices, and pepper. Top tomato halves with fresh basil and **Melba Toast Crumbs**. Bake or broil 5-7 minutes until lightly browned and serve.

Sweet and Spicy Apple Chard

Ingredients
1 1/2 cups chard, chopped
1 apple, diced
3/4 cup water
2 slices lemon with rind
1/2 teaspoon garam masala
1/4 teaspoon curry
Stevia to taste
Pinch of salt

Makes 1 serving
(1 fruit, 1 vegetable)

2 grams protein

0 grams fat

150 calories

Sauté chard, apple, lemon, and spices in water until chard is tender and liquid is reduced, approximately 10 minutes. Add Stevia to taste and serve.

Desserts

Broiled Vanilla Grapefruit

Strawberry Cheesecake

Gingered Apple Pudding

Apples with Caramel Dip

Apples with Cinnamon Pie Dip

Orange Coconut Sticks

Green Tea Strawberry Sorbet

Apple Meringue Pie

Fruit with Chocolate Sauce

Cinnamon Meringue Puffs

Strawberry Pie

Broiled Vanilla Grapefruit

Ingredients
1/2 grapefruit, in segments
1 teaspoon lemon juice
1 teaspoon ginger, fresh grated
1/8 teaspoon vanilla powder
Vanilla or French Toast / Maple Flavor drops to taste (optional)

▶ Arrange slices in brûlée or small baking dish. Sprinkle with vanilla powder, ginger, and Flavor drops. Broil for approximately 3-5 minutes. Serve warm.

Variations: Top with spiced and sweetened **Melba Toast Crumbs**.

Makes 1 serving
(1 fruit)

1 gram protein

0 grams fat

55 calories

Strawberry Cheesecake

Ingredients
4 large strawberries (plus 1 for topping)
100 grams nonfat cottage cheese
1 tablespoon milk
5 Cheesecake Flavor drops or to taste
Stevia to taste

▶ Puree strawberries with cottage cheese, milk, Stevia, and Flavor drops. Serve chilled.

Variations: Freeze for a frozen treat.

Makes 1 serving
(1 protein, 1 fruit)

17.5 grams protein

.5 gram fat

115 calories

PHASE 3
MODIFICATIONS:
Substitute mixed berries, top with whipped cream or serve as a dip with fruit.

Gingered Apple Pudding

Ingredients
1 apple, cut into wedges
3/4 cup water
1 tablespoon apple water from cooking
1 teaspoon lemon juice
1/2 teaspoon apple cider vinegar
1/4 teaspoon powdered ginger
5 French Toast / Maple Flavor drops
Stevia to taste

Makes 1 serving
(1 fruit)

1 gram protein

0 grams fat

92 calories

Sauté apple in 3/4 cup water for approximately 5 minutes. Add spices and puree apples with liquid ingredients in a blender or food processor.

Apples with Caramel Dip

Ingredients
100 grams nonfat cottage cheese
1 apple, sliced
Stevia (English Toffee) to taste
7-10 Caramel Flavor drops to taste

Makes 1 serving
(1 protein, 1 fruit)

17.5 grams protein

.5 gram fat

175 calories

Puree cottage cheese with Stevia and flavorings in blender or food processor until smooth and creamy. Chill and serve with apple slices.

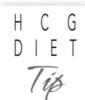

HCG DIET *Tip*

Avoid artificial sweeteners and additives. Choosing a natural, calorie-free sweetener like Stevia is healthier for your body and won't stall your weight loss.

Apples with Cinnamon Pie Dip

Ingredients
1 apple, sliced
100 grams nonfat cottage cheese
1/4 cup water
1/2 teaspoon pumpkin
Stevia to taste (English Toffee or Vanilla)

Makes 1 serving
(1 protein, 1 fruit)

18 grams protein

5 grams fat

178 calories

> Puree cottage cheese and spices with water in a blender until smooth and creamy. Serve with sliced apples.

Orange Coconut Sticks

Ingredients
1 orange, in segments
1 tablespoon lemon juice
1/8 teaspoon vanilla powder
8-10 drops Coconut Flavor drops (1-2 drops per segment)
Stevia to taste

Makes 1 serving
(1 fruit)

1 gram protein

0 grams fat

67 calories

PHASE 3
MODIFICATIONS: Roll in
2 tablespoons coconut.

> Segment orange. Roll in lemon juice, vanilla powder, and Stevia. Add 1-2 Flavor drops per segment. Place in a plastic bag and freeze.

Green Tea Strawberry Sorbet

Ingredients
3/4 cup iced green tea
3 large frozen strawberries
1 tablespoon milk (optional)
1 teaspoon lemon juice
7 French Vanilla Flavor drops (optional)
3 ice cubes
Stevia to taste

Makes 1 serving
(1 fruit)

0 protein

0 grams fat

20 calories

> Brew tea and allow to chill in refrigerator. Add strawberries, lemon juice, Flavor drops, Stevia, and ice cubes. Puree in a blender and serve.

Apple Meringue Pie

Ingredients

1 apple, minced or cubed

1 egg white (eat the rest of an egg serving to complete a
   protein for that meal)

2 tablespoons water

1 teaspoon lemon juice

1/2 teaspoon apple cider vinegar

1/8 teaspoon cinnamon

1/8 teaspoon ginger

Pinch of nutmeg

Pinch of vanilla powder

Stevia (English Toffee or Vanilla) to taste

Makes 1 serving
(1 fruit, 1 protein)

4 grams protein

0 grams fat

112 calories

> Mince apples and mix in half of spices. Add lemon juice, apple cider
> vinegar and water, and mix to combine flavors. Bake at 375 degrees
> for 10 minutes. Remove apple pie and allow to cool slightly. Whip egg
> white to firm peaks. Add Stevia and vanilla powder. Top apple pie with
> meringue. Dust with additional spices such as cinnamon and ginger
> and broil for 3-5 minutes until lightly browned.

Fruit with Chocolate Sauce

Your choice of allowed fruit

Chocolate Sauce

Ingredients

1 teaspoon defatted cocoa powder

Chocolate Flavor drops (optional)

2 tablespoons water

1 tablespoon milk

1/4 teaspoon vanilla powder

Stevia to taste

Makes 1 serving
(1 fruit)

1 gram protein

0 grams fat

<10 calories plus the
calories in the fruit

> Heat water and milk. Dissolve cocoa, vanilla, Flavor drops, and
> Stevia into milk mixture and stir until creamy. Drizzle over fresh
> fruit or dip and enjoy.

Cinnamon Meringue Puffs

Ingredients
1 egg white
1/2 teaspoon cinnamon
Pinch of vanilla powder
Powdered Stevia to taste

▶ Preheat oven to 250 degrees. Whip meringue until stiff. Whip in cinnamon, Stevia, and vanilla powder. Drop cookies onto parchment paper on a cookie sheet and bake for one hour.

Variations: Experiment with different Flavor drops, spices, etc.

Makes a partial serving
(1 protein)
(complete a protein
serving by eating 1 whole
egg and 2 egg whites
at the time you enjoy
meringue cookies)

3.5 grams protein
0 grams fat
19 calories

Strawberry Pie

Ingredients
5 large strawberries
1 cup fennel, soft cooked (to make 1/2 cup pureed)
1 serving **Melba Toast Crumbs** (optional)
2 tablespoons lemon juice
2 tablespoons water
1/4 teaspoon defatted cocoa or vanilla powder (optional)
Stevia to taste (English Toffee or Vanilla works best)

▶ Preheat oven to 400 degrees. Steam fennel until tender and puree. Add strawberries to 1/2 cup pureed fennel, lemon juice, water and Stevia and puree the mixture together. Fold into brûlée or small baking dish. Mix **Melba Toast Crumbs** with Stevia and defatted cocoa or vanilla. Top strawberry mixture with **Melba Toast Crumbs** and bake for 20-25 minutes until bubbly and lightly browned on top.

Variations: Add a pinch of cocoa powder, cinnamon or other spices to pie.

Makes 1 serving
(1 protein, 1 vegetable,
1 Melba toast)

2 grams protein
0 grams fat
78 calories

HCG
DIET
Tip   *Add fruit flavored Stevia drops to sweeten your favorite Desserts or Beverages.*

Beverages

Citrus Freeze

Ginger Ale

Chai Smoothie

Lemon Berry Sorbet

Cucumber Lemonade

Chocolate Coconut Freeze

Strawberry Colada

Sparkling Orange Cranberry Tea

Mint Julep (non-alcoholic)

Chocolate Strawberry Shake

Citrus Freeze

Ingredients
4 frozen grapefruit spears (eat the rest of your 1/2 grapefruit to
  complete a fruit serving)
1 tablespoon lemon juice
8 Orange Flavor drops (optional) or Orange or Vanilla Stevia (optional)
Stevia to taste
3 ice cubes

Makes 1 serving
(1 fruit)

.5 gram protein

0 grams fat

40 calories

▶ Puree ingredients in blender and serve.

Variations: Substitute 5 frozen orange segments.

Ginger Ale

Ingredients
Ginger sauce to taste
6 ounces sparkling mineral water
Ice

Makes 1 serving

0 protein

0 grams fat

>5 calories

Ginger Sauce
Ingredients
1 cup water
5 medium slices ginger, fresh, peeled
1 teaspoon vanilla powder
Stevia to taste

▶ Combine ginger sauce ingredients in a small saucepan. Cook until
  liquid is reduced by half. Allow to cool then chill in the refrigerator.
  Remove ginger slices. Add 2 ounces **Ginger Sauce** to 6 ounces of
  sparkling mineral water and pour over ice.

Chai Smoothie

Ingredients
1 cup cold brewed Chai tea
1 tablespoon nonfat milk
French Vanilla Flavor drops or English Toffee Stevia
Stevia to taste
3 ice cubes

Makes 1 serving
<1 gram protein
<1 grams fat
3 calories

 Puree ingredients in blender and serve.

Variations: You can substitute any flavorful herbal tea for this recipe. Orange, coconut, and cranberry flavored teas are delicious served this way.

Lemon Berry Sorbet

Ingredients
Any variety berry tea (bagged)
1/4 cup hot water
2 frozen lemon slices, without rind
2 frozen strawberries (eat 3-4 additional strawberries
   to complete a fruit serving)
1/8 teaspoon vanilla powder (substitute Vanilla Stevia or
   Vanilla Flavor drops)
Pinch of lemon zest
Stevia to taste
Ice

Makes 1 serving (1 fruit)
1 gram protein
0 grams fat
12 calories

Brew tea in hot water. Allow to cool then puree with ice, frozen fruits, Stevia, and flavorings. Serve iced or freeze into pops.

HCG DIET Tip *Enjoy a delicious iced blended Beverage on the HCG Phase to help with hunger. An herbal tea or Stevia sweetened drink has no calories and tastes delicious.*

Cucumber Lemonade

Ingredients
1/2 large cucumber
Juice of 1/4 lemon
Stevia to taste
Ice cubes

Makes 1 serving
(1 vegetable)

1 gram protein

0 grams fat

22 calories

> Combine ingredients and puree in blender. Serve over ice or as a light tangy drink.

Variation: Substitute orange flavored Stevia and/or fresh grated ginger.

Chocolate Coconut Freeze

Ingredients
3/4 cup chilled coffee
1 tablespoon milk (optional)
1/2 teaspoon defatted cocoa
5 drops Coconut Flavor drops
Stevia to taste
4 ice cubes

Makes 1 serving

<1 gram protein

0 grams fat

<5 calories

> Puree coffee and other ingredients with ice and serve.

Strawberry Colada

Ingredients
3 sliced strawberries, frozen
1/2 cup water (substitute coconut tea)
1 tablespoon milk (optional)
1 teaspoon lemon juice
5-7 Coconut Flavor drops or to taste (optional)
Stevia to taste
4 ice cubes

Makes 1 serving
(1 fruit)

<1 gram protein

<1 gram fat

20 calories

PHASE 3
MODIFICATIONS: Add
one shot of rum.

> Blend ingredients in blender and serve.

Sparkling Orange Cranberry Tea

Ingredients
1 bag cranberry tea
1/4 cup hot water
6 ounces sparkling water
Lemon slices
Pinch of orange zest
Stevia to taste
Ice

Makes 1 serving
0 protein
0 grams fat
0 calories

> Brew cranberry tea in hot water. Allow to cool. Add Stevia, orange zest, sparkling water, and lemon slices. Serve over ice.

Mint Julep (non-alcoholic)

Ingredients
Mint leaves, crushed
Juice of 2 lemon wedges
1/4 cup water
1 lemon slice
1/2 cup water (sparkling or flat)
Stevia to taste
Ice

Makes 1 serving
0 protein
0 grams fat
0 calories

PHASE 3
MODIFICATION: Add a
shot of bourbon.

> Lightly warm water, lemon juice, Stevia, and crushed mint in a small saucepan until flavors are infused. Allow to cool. Add sparkling water then serve over ice with a lemon wedge.

Chocolate Strawberry Shake

Ingredients
5 large strawberries
1 tablespoon milk (optional)
1/4-1/2 teaspoon defatted cocoa
Chocolate Stevia to taste
4 ice cubes

Makes 1 serving
(1 fruit)
1 gram protein
<1 gram fat
35 calories

> Puree ingredients in a blender and serve. You can also pour into molds and serve as an ice pop or sorbet.

Conclusion

The HCG Diet is changing lives around the world, and I'm so thrilled that you have discovered the incredible benefits and rapid weight loss from this program. I sincerely hope that the information and recipes in this cookbook inspire and help you along the way as you lose all the weight you desire with the HCG Diet. It is my goal with this cookbook to bring some fun and flavor into your life and make it a little easier to stick to this program. Enjoy the amazing changes taking place in your body. I encourage you to take this opportunity, while on this program and beyond, to make shifts in how you choose the food you eat and feel about your body.

As someone who has struggled with weight my entire life right up until I discovered this program, I understand the challenges you face and the thrill of finally finding a diet that actually works! And offers lasting results!

I speak from experience that this diet is a miracle and I know that the journey you are on with the HCG Diet can truly change your life. I thank you for allowing me, in some small way, to be part of your transformation.

I wish you the very best in your life and all the success in the world.

Tammy Skye

Tammy Skye

ABOUT THE AUTHOR

Tammy Skye is a fellow HCG Dieter who has lost almost 60 pounds with the amazing HCG Diet. She has a medical background as a Physical Therapist Assistant and has an avid interest in alternative medicine, natural health and healing, and nutrition. She considers herself a dedicated "foodie" and loves to create flavorful, fun dishes using unusual ingredients, unique combinations, and healthy recipe versions of favorite "comfort" foods.

She wrote her first book, "The HCG Diet Gourmet Cookbook, Volume 1" in 2007 and released it as an e-book to a handful of HCG Dieters. She published the book in print in April of 2010. It is her mission to help educate and share her recipes and information about the original HCG Diet Program with other dieters to help them be successful and maintain their weight loss.

Testimonials

"I LOVE LOVE LOVE **The HCG Diet Gourmet Cookbook**! The recipes are really really good and made what could have been a very bland diet an enjoyable one instead. I have reached my weight loss goals and Tammy's first HCG Cookbook truly made all the difference in my HCG diet journey."

— Darlene - CA

"Your **HCG Diet Gourmet Cookbook** was a life saver for me. After I bought it, I had no trouble with variety in my HCG Diet meals. Can't wait till the next book comes out!"

— Linda

"Our patients love the cookbook and are able to set up meal plans by just following what is in the book. I would recommend for anyone interested in doing the HCG diet program that he/she get a copy of Tammy Skye's **The HCG Diet Gourmet Cookbook**. It will be a great asset to their weight loss program."

—Kenneth E. Baird, MD, The Baird Family Clinic - TX

Other Books by Tammy Skye

The HCG Diet Gourmet Cookbook, Volume 1: Over 200 "Low Calorie" Recipes for the HCG Phase

www.hcgrecipes.com

The HCG Diet Gourmet Cookbook Volume 3 "The Stabilization Phase" (Phase 3 or P3)

Enjoy these delicious Phase 3 Stabilization recipes to help you manage your weight and reset your metabolism on the HCG Diet. Featuring a wide variety of starch and sugar free entrees, appetizers, soups and salads, and decadent desserts as you transition to the *Stabilization Phase* of the HCG Diet.

www.hcgrecipes.com

Libro de Recetes de la Dieta HCG Vol. 1

(*The HCG Diet Gourmet Cookbook Volume 1 - Spanish translation*)

www.hcgrecetas.com

The Fibernoodle Cookbook

Featuring the amazing, calorie free, pure fiber, Shirataki noodles from Japan. These delicious recipes feature many homestyle favorites, Italian pasta recipes, Asian noodle dishes, and more. The recipes are prepared without sugar or starch and are easily adapted to the *Stabilization Phase* (Phase 3 or P3) of the HCG Diet.

www.fibernoodlecookbook.com

The Coffee, Tea, Sugar Free Cookbook

Featuring delicious specialty coffee and tea drink recipes using all natural Stevia.

www.coffeeteasugarfree.com

HCG Diet Stories

Inspiring true stories of real HCG Dieters (with co-author Lynne Scott).

www.hcgdietstories.com

PRIVACY NOTE: We will never share your e-mail address. You can easily request to be removed from our list at any time. Instructions are included with every e-mail we send.

Sign up to be on the list for Free Gifts and Big Discounts when new books are released

www.hcgrecipes.com/updates

RESOURCES AND LINKS

RECOMMENDED READING

Pounds and Inches: A New Approach to Obesity

The original HCG Diet program and book by Dr. A.T.W. Simeons. You can find a copy of this amazing book on my website.

www.hcgrecipes.com.

The Weight Loss Cure They Don't Want You to Know About

The revolutionary book by Kevin Trudeau that discusses the HCG Diet in detail with additional nutrition and wellness recommendations for healthy living.

www.naturalcures.com (can be purchased at most bookstores)

HCG Diet Made Simple

An invaluable guide for HCG Dieters by Harmony Clearwater Grace that offers step by step advice and a wealth of valuable information and resources to help you lose weight and be successful with the HCG Diet.

www.hcgdietmadesimplebook.com

Visit the HCGrecipes blog for more HCG Diet tips, health and wellness information, and recipes at www.hcgrecipes.com/blog.

Make a difference and DEMAND a natural alternative to sugar and artificial sweeteners. Ask for Stevia at your favorite restaurant or coffee shop today.

www.askforstevia.com

Dear Dieter,

To help you with your diet, I've prepared some special free gifts just for you. You can access your bonus HCG Diet tools here:

http://pages.hcgrecipes.com/secret-stash-5

Scan the code below with your smartphone for more info, updates, discounts, and more or go to www.hcgrecipes.com.

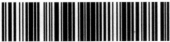

11907880R00102

Made in the USA
Middletown, DE
15 November 2018